DEFENDING THE U.S. AIR TRANSPORTATION SYSTEM AGAINST CHEMICAL AND BIOLOGICAL THREATS

Committee on Assessment of Security Technologies for Transportation

National Materials Advisory Board

Division on Engineering and Physical Sciences

NATIONAL RESEARCH COUNCIL
OF THE NATIONAL ACADEMIES

THE NATIONAL ACADEMIES PRESS
Washington, D.C.
www.nap.edu

THE NATIONAL ACADEMIES PRESS 500 Fifth Street, N.W. Washington, DC 20001

NOTICE: The project that is the subject of this report was approved by the Governing Board of the National Research Council, whose members are drawn from the councils of the National Academy of Sciences, the National Academy of Engineering, and the Institute of Medicine. The members of the committee responsible for the report were chosen for their special competences and with regard for appropriate balance.

This study was supported by Contract No. DTFA03-99-C-00006 between the National Academy of Sciences and the Transportation Security Administration. Any opinions, findings, conclusions, or recommendations expressed in this publication are those of the author(s) and do not necessarily reflect the views of the agency that provided support for the project.

A limited number of copies of this report are available from the National Materials Advisory Board, 500 Fifth Street, N.W., Keck WS932, Washington, DC 20001; (202) 334-3505 or (202) 334-3718; Internet, http://www.nas.edu/nmab.

Additional copies of this report are available from the National Academies Press, 500 Fifth Street, N.W., Lockbox 285, Washington, DC 20055; (800) 624-6242 or (202) 334-3313 (in the Washington metropolitan area); Internet, http://www.nap.edu.

International Standard Book Number 0-309-10074-7

Printed in the United States of America

THE NATIONAL ACADEMIES

Advisers to the Nation on Science, Engineering, and Medicine

The **National Academy of Sciences** is a private, nonprofit, self-perpetuating society of distinguished scholars engaged in scientific and engineering research, dedicated to the furtherance of science and technology and to their use for the general welfare. Upon the authority of the charter granted to it by the Congress in 1863, the Academy has a mandate that requires it to advise the federal government on scientific and technical matters. Dr. Ralph J. Cicerone is president of the National Academy of Sciences.

The **National Academy of Engineering** was established in 1964, under the charter of the National Academy of Sciences, as a parallel organization of outstanding engineers. It is autonomous in its administration and in the selection of its members, sharing with the National Academy of Sciences the responsibility for advising the federal government. The National Academy of Engineering also sponsors engineering programs aimed at meeting national needs, encourages education and research, and recognizes the superior achievements of engineers. Dr. Wm. A. Wulf is president of the National Academy of Engineering.

The **Institute of Medicine** was established in 1970 by the National Academy of Sciences to secure the services of eminent members of appropriate professions in the examination of policy matters pertaining to the health of the public. The Institute acts under the responsibility given to the National Academy of Sciences by its congressional charter to be an adviser to the federal government and, upon its own initiative, to identify issues of medical care, research, and education. Dr. Harvey V. Fineberg is president of the Institute of Medicine.

The **National Research Council** was organized by the National Academy of Sciences in 1916 to associate the broad community of science and technology with the Academy's purposes of furthering knowledge and advising the federal government. Functioning in accordance with general policies determined by the Academy, the Council has become the principal operating agency of both the National Academy of Sciences and the National Academy of Engineering in providing services to the government, the public, and the scientific and engineering communities. The Council is administered jointly by both Academies and the Institute of Medicine. Dr. Ralph J. Cicerone and Dr. Wm. A. Wulf are chair and vice chair, respectively, of the National Research Council.

www.national-academies.org

COMMITTEE ON ASSESSMENT OF SECURITY TECHNOLOGIES FOR TRANSPORTATION

JAMES F. O'BRYON, *Chair*, The O'Bryon Group, Belair, Maryland
SANDRA L. HYLAND, *Vice Chair*, Tokyo Electron Technology Center, Albany, New York
CHERYL A. BITNER, AAI Corporation, Phoenix, Maryland
DONALD E. BROWN, University of Virginia, Charlottesville
JOHN B. DALY, Consultant, Arlington, Virginia
COLIN G. DRURY, State University of New York at Buffalo
PATRICK GRIFFIN, Sandia National Laboratories, Albuquerque, New Mexico
JIRI JANATA, Georgia Institute of Technology, Atlanta
HARRY E. MARTZ, JR., Lawrence Livermore National Laboratory, Livermore, California
RICHARD McGEE, Army Research Laboratory, Aberdeen Proving Ground, Maryland
RICHARD L. ROWE, Safeview, Saratoga, California
ERIC R. SCHWARTZ, The Boeing Company, Huntington Beach, California
MICHAEL STORY, Consultant, Los Gatos, California
H. BRUCE WALLACE, ORSA Corporation, Aberdeen, Maryland

Staff

JAMES KILLIAN, Study Director
TERI G. THOROWGOOD, Administrative Coordinator

NATIONAL MATERIALS ADVISORY BOARD

Staff

Preface

The Committee on Assessment of Security Technologies for Transportation was appointed by the National Research Council (NRC) in response to a request from the Transportation Security Administration (TSA) for a study of technologies to protect the nation's air transportation system from terrorist attacks. The committee judged that the best way to provide a timely response would be to produce a series of short reports on promising technologies, focusing on specific topics of greatest interest to the sponsor. This is the second of four such topical reports, all of which focus on air transportation security.[1] The committee believes that the air transportation environment provides a test case for the deployment of security technologies that could subsequently be used to protect other transportation modes as well.

The discovery in February 2004 of the biological poison ricin in a Senate office building in Washington, D.C., highlights the fact that the terrorist's arsenal now includes not only the all-too-familiar weapons such as small arms and explosives, but also chemical and biological agents. This expanding arsenal demands that policy makers and transportation authorities consider the deployment of new defensive technologies to respond to the new threats. In this report, the committee explores defensive strategies that could be used to protect air transportation spaces (specifically, airport terminals and aircraft) against attack with chemical or biological agents and makes recommendations with respect to the role of TSA in implementing these strategies.

The committee acknowledges the speakers from government and industry who took the time to share their ideas and experiences in briefings at the committee's meetings. The committee would like to offer special thanks to Jiri Janata and Richard Rowe, who were the major contributors to the writing of this report. The following former committee members also greatly assisted the work of the current committee through their participation in many of its activities: Thomas S. Hartwick, chair through May 31, 2005; Len Limmer, consultant; and Elizabeth H. Slate, Medical University of South Carolina. Finally, the committee acknowledges the contributions to the completion of this report from National Materials Advisory Board director Gary Fischman, consultant Greg Eyring, and NRC staff members James Killian and Teri Thorowgood.

James F. O'Bryon, *Chair*
Sandra L. Hyland, *Vice Chair*
Committee on Assessment of
Security Technologies for Transportation

---

[1]The first report was *Opportunities to Improve Airport Passenger Screening with Mass Spectrometry* (The National Academies Press, Washington, D.C., 2004). Topics to be addressed in future reports are millimeter-wave imaging for detection of explosives and data fusion and integration for airport terminals.

Acknowledgment of Reviewers

This report has been reviewed in draft form by individuals chosen for their diverse perspectives and technical expertise, in accordance with procedures approved by the National Research Council's Report Review Committee. The purpose of this independent review is to provide candid and critical comments that will assist the institution in making its published report as sound as possible and to ensure that the report meets institutional standards for objectivity, evidence, and responsiveness to the study charge. The review comments and draft manuscript remain confidential to protect the integrity of the deliberative process. We wish to thank the following individuals for their review of this report:

Raymond H. Bittel, The Boeing Company,
John Brockman, Sandia National Laboratories,
Philip E. Coyle III, Science Strategies,
Susanna P. Gordon, Sandia National Laboratories,
Mohamed Sofi Ibrahim, USAMRIID,
Edwin P. Przybylowicz, Eastman Kodak Co., retired, and
R. Paul Schaudies, Science Applications International Corporation.

Although the reviewers listed above have provided many constructive comments and suggestions, they were not asked to endorse the conclusions or recommendations, nor did they see the final draft of the report before its release. The review of this report was overseen by R. Stephen Berry, University of Chicago. Appointed by the National Research Council, he was responsible for making certain that an independent examination of this report was carried out in accordance with institutional procedures and that all review comments were carefully considered. Responsibility for the final content of this report rests solely with the authoring committee and the institution.

Contents

Figures and Tables

FIGURES

TABLES

Acronyms

DARPA	Defense Advanced Research Projects Agency
DHS	Department of Homeland Security
DOD	Department of Defense
DOE	Department of Energy
ECS	Environmental Control System
HEPA	high-efficiency particulate air
HVAC	heating, ventilation, and air conditioning
LCT_{50}	lethal concentration of toxin at which 50 percent of test animals are killed
NRC	National Research Council
NSF	National Science Foundation
PFA	probability of false alarms
POD	probability of detection
PROACT	Protective and Response Options for Airport Counter-Terrorism
PROTECT	Program for Response Options and Technology Enhancements for Chemical/Biological Terrorism
SARS	severe acute respiratory syndrome
SBCCOM	Soldier Biological and Chemical Command
SFIA	San Francisco International Airport
TSA	Transportation Security Administration
TSWG	Technical Support Working Group
UV	ultraviolet

Executive Summary

Historically, most terrorist attacks on civilian targets have involved the use of firearms or explosives, and current defensive strategies are aimed at preventing attacks perpetrated by such means. However, the use of the nerve agent sarin in 1995 to attack the Tokyo subway system, the use of the U.S. mail in 2001 to distribute letters containing anthrax spores, and the discovery in 2004 of the biological toxin ricin in U.S. Senate Office Buildings in Washington, D.C., demonstrate that chemical and biological agents have been added to terrorists' arsenals. Attacks involving chemical/biological agents are of great concern, not only because of the potential for mass casualties but also because there is no strategy or technology fielded today that can respond adequately to this threat. As the United States and other countries reassess the security measures they have in place to prevent or defend against such attacks (particularly in areas where large numbers of people gather and then widely disperse), the risks to the air transportation system as a primary target become clear.

While potential attacks on all modes of transportation are of concern, the Committee on Assessment of Security Technologies for Transportation believes that the U.S. air transportation system continues to have a high priority for counterterrorism resources, both because of its economic importance and because of the intensified public perception of risk following the September 11, 2001, attacks. The air transportation system can also serve as a testbed for the development of defensive technologies and strategies that can subsequently be applied to other transportation modes.

Finding 1: The U.S. air transportation system is an attractive target for attacks with chemical or biological weapons, yet no federal agency has been assigned clear responsibility for developing a strategy for defense against such attacks.

The large numbers of people gathered in air terminals—perpetually coming and going—provide anonymity to the terrorist, and the fact that most passengers carry luggage makes the detection of threat agents concealed in luggage more difficult. The rapid dispersal of passengers from air terminals to destinations around the world means that those who become infected with communicable diseases could spread the diseases widely in a short time, a situation that was demonstrated in 2003 in the case of the severe acute respiratory syndrome (SARS) virus. Finally, a chemical/biological attack on the U.S. air transportation system would raise the already high level of public anxiety about travel risks and would likely result in significant economic disruption.

Considerable research on defensive concepts against chemical/biological attacks is being funded by the Department of Homeland Security (DHS), the Department of Defense (DOD), the Department of Energy's (DOE's) national laboratories, the Technical Support Working Group (TSWG),[1] the Centers for Disease Control and Prevention, and other agencies. The DHS has supported preliminary studies aimed at improving the defenses of airports against chemical/biological attacks, but the future funding and scope of these efforts remain in doubt. Within DHS, the Transportation Security Administration (TSA), which has the lead in defending the system against concealed weapons and explosives, has not been assigned responsibility for leading the defense against chemical/biological attack.

Recommendation 1: The Transportation Security Administration, with its responsibility for the federal oversight of security operations at U.S. airports, should integrate strategies for defense against chemical/biological attacks into its broader security plan for protecting the U.S. air transportation system. The line of authority and

[1] The Technical Support Working Group is the U.S. national forum that identifies, prioritizes, and coordinates interagency and international research and development requirements for combating terrorism.

accountability for implementing these strategies should be clearly defined.

Air transportation spaces range from very large spaces (e.g., terminals) to very small spaces (e.g., aircraft), with unique characteristics that will help shape defensive strategies for the respective areas. For instance, given the likely dissemination of threat agents through the air in a chemical/biological attack, the air-handling systems in these spaces are likely to be a particularly important factor in the mitigation of the impact of any attack. Because of its ongoing work to address threats from explosives in air transportation environments, TSA is the agency most knowledgeable about the unique characteristics of these spaces; it is well positioned to extend this work to encompass chemical/biological threats.[2]

Finding 2: No specific strategies, approaches, or procedures have been developed to defend the U.S. air transportation system against chemical/biological attacks.

Plausible scenarios for terrorist chemical/biological attacks include point releases of plumes of threat agents in various locations in a terminal or on air transportation vehicles, or releases directly into the air-handling systems of these spaces. Many different chemicals or biological organisms might be used—each with its own physical, chemical, and biological properties, which would influence the dispersal of the agent and the exposure of potential victims. Attacks might involve fast-acting agents (generally chemicals), causing victims' symptoms to appear within seconds to minutes, or slower-acting agents (generally biological toxins or microorganisms), exposure to which occurs rapidly, although symptoms may not appear until after a delay of hours to days. The latter include infectious as well as noncommunicable viral and bacterial agents.

The DHS has funded preliminary studies to elaborate specific chemical/biological threat vectors, to increase understanding of airflows, and to demonstrate chemical/biological detection systems in several terminals and boarding areas in two airports (San Francisco International Airport and Albuquerque Airport). The DHS has also conducted an exercise in which the many airport decision makers (e.g., in areas of operations, security, fire control and prevention, public health and safety, and environmental issues) come together to try to formulate a coordinated response to a simulated chemical/biological attack. Such studies and exercises are valuable and should result in useful guidance that can help many airports to begin to think about their own response plans. However, the work thus far is preliminary and of limited scope, and TSA itself appears to have had little involvement. Although TSA does participate in interagency groups that address homeland security issues (e.g., the Technical Support Working Group), the specific requirements of air transportation systems have not been given a high priority, according to briefings to the committee by TSA personnel who have attended these meetings.

Recommendation 2: The Transportation Security Administration, in collaboration with other appropriate entities within the Department of Homeland Security,[3] should create a high-level task force to perform the following functions:

- **Create a validated threat assessment document for air transportation spaces and keep it updated;**
- **Take advantage of ongoing research aimed at the development of models of the airflow within aircraft, terminals, and so forth, based on empirical studies of specific facilities, and explore the dispersal of chemical/biological simulants under various release scenarios;**
- **Create guidance to help air transportation facilities develop a threat defense strategy; and**
- **Determine unique air transportation requirements for dealing with chemical/biological threats and coordinate closely with other agencies that are active in the chemical/biological threats area to ensure that these requirements are given visibility in their programs.**

This defensive strategy should include elements such as the following: contingency plans for responding to scenarios involving the release of various threat agents, clearly defined areas of responsibility for key decision makers, training for first-responders, plans for the evacuation of potential victims of attacks, plans for the isolation of contaminated areas, strategies for the early treatment of exposed individuals, timely remediation of affected areas, and rapid restoration of flight operations to ensure minimal adverse impact to the air traffic system.

The scale of the response to a chemical/biological attack must be commensurate with the level of confidence that an attack has indeed taken place. This is particularly important for attacks involving slow-acting agents, in which a detector alarm may be the only indication that an attack has occurred. For cases in which the detector has a relatively high rate of false-positive alarms, there may be a range of "low-regret" responses that could provide some measure of protection without producing the degree of disruption that might be justified if the certainty of attack were higher. An example of a low-regret response might be choosing to shut down the heating, ventilation, and air conditioning (HVAC) system to reduce the potential spread of agent while the validity of an

[2]The federal security directors at all major airports (these individuals are TSA employees) have operational control for security and are charged with organizing and implementing crisis management response plans.

[3]Currently, the DHS entity with the most knowledge and experience in this area is the Science and Technology Directorate.

alarm is being assessed, rather than immediately evacuating an air terminal. This response could be augmented, again without causing disruption to airport operations, by dynamically fast-acting HVAC pressure control in which air spaces adjacent to the potentially contaminated air space would be positively pressured to protect them from any hazardous agents.

Finding 3: Many alternative chemical/biological detection technologies are being investigated in university, industry, and government laboratories, and various military prototype systems have been developed; however, it is very difficult to independently evaluate all of the performance claims for these technologies.

A staggering number of papers are published each year in the literature on various candidate chemical/biological detection systems. Researchers and manufacturers make diverse claims of detection limits, sensitivity, false-alarm rates, and robustness for these systems. The committee believes that in many cases, researchers emphasize the strengths of their particular detection systems while minimizing or ignoring their flaws. This practice makes it virtually impossible to evaluate the likely performance of a detection system in real-world air transportation environments.

The committee received briefings on numerous research programs around the country aimed at developing various chemical/biological detection systems. Several of these show promise, including some evaluated by an earlier NRC panel[4] and one (mass spectrometry) evaluated previously by this committee. However, each technology appears to require substantial development and verification testing before it could be deployed in an airport or other transportation space.

Recommendation 3: The Transportation Security Administration should keep abreast of ongoing research on chemical/biological detector technologies without starting an in-house research and development activity. Rather, it should seek to leverage the research programs of other agencies, and it should consider supporting a vendor-independent testing capability in order to verify performance claims made for chemical/biological detection systems.

The primary technology mission and expertise of TSA's laboratories and personnel involve the detection of weapons and concealed explosives. The TSA does not have the resources or expertise to develop detection and identification systems for chemical/biological agents. However, TSA's technology-monitoring effort might involve funding a third party to survey the spectrum of detection technologies in order to identify those that might be most appropriate for the air transportation environment.

The TSA should maintain close liaison with other agencies (e.g., DOD, DOE, and the TSWG) to leverage their chemical/biological research efforts and to ensure that air transportation requirements are given a high priority. The TSA should also consider supporting an independent body to develop test criteria and to conduct standard tests to evaluate the performance of chemical/biological detection systems and to verify the claims of prospective manufacturers. Such an independent testing body would benefit the ongoing research efforts of many government agencies.

Finding 4: Although the rapid detection of a chemical/biological attack and identification of the agent used are worthwhile objectives, a defensive strategy that depends exclusively on a detection-system alarm before action is taken (i.e., employment of a "detect and react" strategy) has several serious limitations.

In an attack with fast-acting agents, the chemicals would reach the victims and begin producing symptoms in approximately the same amount of time that these same chemicals would take to reach and produce a response from a technology-based detector. Thus, the best "detector" of a fast-acting agent may be visual evidence that people are collapsing or behaving in unusual ways. Visual recognition of symptoms cannot be relied on to detect delayed-acting chemical agents or biotoxins (which may not produce symptoms for several hours), and here chemical-detection systems may offer more promise, provided their cost and performance are acceptable.

For the detection of slow-acting biological agents (which may not produce symptoms for several days), the system response time would depend on the frequency of sampling and analysis. The frequency of sampling and analysis would be determined by factors such as the cost of the assay, the frequency with which critical reagents need to be replaced, the robustness of the detector, and so on. The minimum response time would be determined by the time required to collect a sample, prepare it for analysis, conduct the assay, and report the results. In the event of an alarm from a detector with a significant false-alarm rate, additional time would be required to determine its validity and to decide on an appropriate response.

The lengthy response time of such a "detect and react" approach might make it impractical for mitigating the immediate impacts of slow-acting agent attack in the air transportation environment (where passenger residence times are about 1 hour). It could, however, have benefits such as enabling subsequent notification of passengers regarding possible exposures, facilitating forensic investigations, and so on.

[4]National Research Council, *Sensor Systems for Biological Agent Attacks: Protecting Buildings and Military Bases*, Washington, D.C.: The National Academies Press, 2005.

Recommendation 4: Given the limitations of sensor- and assay-based chemical/biological agent detection and identification technologies, the Transportation Security Administration should pursue a baseline defensive strategy against chemical/biological attacks that does not depend solely on the technological detection of threat agents to initiate action. Such a strategy would be based on elements such as the following:

- **Protective and preventative steps and enhanced security;**
- **Improved visual surveillance of air transportation spaces;**
- **The establishment of a separate air supply for spaces that have a critical function (e.g., cockpits, flight-control towers, emergency-response centers); and**
- **Continuous air treatment to neutralize and/or remove agents or contaminants.**

It is the judgment of this committee that the very large number of candidate sensor-based and assay-based detection systems have received a great deal of attention and research money but that none currently has the effectiveness, technical maturity, reliability, sensitivity, and selectivity to many different agents, nor the low cost, needed for deployment in the air transportation environment. In contrast, a variety of existing technologies that do not involve the detection of an agent could prevent or mitigate the consequences of chemical/biological attacks; such technologies are available today and would be arguably less costly to deploy. These "non-technological-detector-based" defensive measures (e.g., air cleaning, better security, better control of airflows) have not received the attention and analysis that the committee believes they deserve. Generally, the committee believes that technologies associated with non-detection-based strategies are nearer term, whereas technologies associated with detection-based strategies (with the exception of video-camera surveillance) are longer term or more speculative. Appropriate protective steps might include ensuring that the air-handling systems inside a terminal are balanced to reduce airflow between regions that could spread chemical and biological agents more rapidly. Enhanced security would include limiting physical access to the intake of air-handling systems—both for terminals and for aircraft on the ground.

To combat attacks with fast-acting agents in the terminals, continuous visual surveillance of densely populated areas and observation of behavior patterns may be as useful as any detector. The TSA should study the feasibility of the widespread deployment of surveillance cameras in populated areas, coupled with behavioral-pattern-recognition software, as an alternative to chemical agent detectors. Such cameras could also provide a dual-use value in improving the overall security environment. In addition, many critical nodes in the air transportation system (control rooms, emergency-response centers, and so on) are supplied with air that is recirculated from publicly accessible areas; this makes them vulnerable to being disabled by the release of chemical/biological agents in these public areas. Thus, it may be prudent to ensure that these critical nodes have an independent air supply and are kept at a positive pressure with respect to surrounding areas.

To combat attacks with slow-acting agents, TSA should study the feasibility of promoting the use of "clean air" systems that would continuously treat the air to remove respirable biological particles and chemicals, both in terminals and in transportation vehicles. This approach might involve a combination of technologies including improved air filtration, ultraviolet irradiation of filters, and/or passing the air through plasma cleaners or other treatment devices. A feasibility study would include the costs (both first cost and maintenance/replacement cost), number and optimum placement of air-cleaning units required, their effectiveness in removing threat agents from the air under various release scenarios, the number of likely exposures prevented, and so on. This defensive strategy would not prevent the exposure of people in the immediate vicinity of a point biological or chemical agent release, but it would limit the exposure of people in surrounding areas resulting from recirculation of the agent through the HVAC system. The provision of "clean air" to passengers would be analogous to municipal water treatment systems that provide clean drinking water to city residents, and it could have the ancillary benefit of reducing the spread of common ills such as cold and flu viruses. Coordination with related programs in other agencies, such as the Immune Building Program of the Defense Advanced Research Projects Agency, should be encouraged.

In conclusion, it appears that, given the need to maintain convenient public access to an efficient air transportation system, a terrorist attack on the system with chemical/biological agents would be difficult to prevent and would likely result in a significant number of casualties. Because there are a very large number of possible chemical and biological agents that might be used in a future terrorist attack and because the specific type of agent to be used would not likely be known in advance, the development and deployment of chemical sensors and bioassays for arbitrarily selected specific agents offer little real protection. By contrast, the deployment of video monitors and/or of biology-based "functional" detectors (analogous to the canary in the mine) that indicate the effects of any fast-acting toxic chemical agents would be beneficial in some attack scenarios. These systems could be deployed in a complementary way with non-detection-based defensive strategies. Thus, preventing or mitigating the overall impact of chemical/biological attacks may depend less on the development of technologies for the detection of threat agents than on prudent protective measures that can be implemented *before such an attack ever takes place*. The TSA should explore the feasibility of these options and should help local authorities and facilities develop contingency plans for responding to chemical/biological attacks on the U.S. air transportation system.

1

Background and Overview

The U.S. air transportation system is an attractive target for terrorists because of the potential for attacks on the system to cause immediate harm and anxiety to large numbers of people, as well as to cause massive economic disruption to the United States and the world. The system is vulnerable because of its mission to provide service to people with a minimum of intrusion on privacy and disruption of access. The detection and mitigation of attacks on air transportation are made more difficult because of the transience of passengers, the small quantity of threat agent that may be required for an effective attack, and the fact that passengers commonly carry baggage, making it relatively easy to conceal threat materials. The September 11, 2001, attacks on the Pentagon and the World Trade Center, in which commercial airliners were used as weapons, also broadened concepts of what constitutes a threat to U.S. assets in general and to the air transportation system in particular.

Based on the history of terrorist attacks, which have mostly involved hijacking and bombing of aircraft, current threat-detection measures have concentrated on detecting weapons or explosives. In the future, terrorist attacks could also involve the use of toxic chemicals, chemical and biological warfare agents, or even radiological and nuclear materials.[1,2]

The government agency charged with responsibility for the implementation of technology for countering such threats is the Transportation Security Administration (TSA) in the Department of Homeland Security. The TSA, and the Federal Aviation Administration before it, have invested extensively in the development and deployment of technological and procedural systems designed to protect the traveling public. In support of its mission, TSA has tasked the National Research Council (NRC) with assessing a variety of technological opportunities for protecting the U.S. transportation system, with a focus on the air transportation system.

STATEMENT OF TASK AND COMMITTEE APPROACH

The TSA has given the NRC the following statement of task for this study:

> This study will explore opportunities for technology to address national needs for transportation security. While the primary role of the committee is to respond to the government's request for assessments in particular applications, the committee may offer advice on specific matters as required. The committee will: (1) identify potential applications for technology in transportation security with a focus on likely threats; (2) evaluate technology approaches to threat detection, effect mitigation, and consequence management; and (3) assess the need for research, development, and deployment to enable implementation of new security technologies. These tasks will be done in the context of current, near-term, and long-term requirements.
>
> The committee will perform the following specific tasks:
>
> 1. Identify potential applications for technology in transportation security with a focus on likely threats derived from threat analyses that drive security system requirements. Review security system developments structured to meet the changing threat environment. Assess government and commercial industry plans designed to address these threats.
>
> 2. Evaluate technology approaches to threat detection, effect mitigation, and consequence management. Delineate the benefits of the insertion of new technologies into existing security systems. Evaluate the trade-offs between effectiveness and cost, including the cost of changing the security system architectures.

---

[1]The President's Homeland Security Department Proposal, available online at http://www.whitehouse.gov/deptofhomeland/bill/index.html. Accessed October 3, 2005.

[2]National Research Council, *Making the Nation Safer: The Role of Science and Technology in Countering Terrorism*, Washington, D.C.: The National Academies Press, 2002.

3. Assess the need for research, development, and deployment to enable implementation of new security technologies. Review and assess the potential benefit of existing and advanced detection technologies, including scanning technologies, sensing technologies, and the use of computer modeling and databases. Review and assess emerging approaches to effect mitigation and consequence management.

An overarching goal of the Committee on Assessment of Security Technologies for Transportation is to provide timely reports that meet TSA's priorities for defeating terrorist threats. The committee judged that this could best be done by issuing a series of short reports on chosen technological applications. In consultation with TSA, the committee selected four topics for review, of which this report is the second:

1. Mass spectrometry for enhanced trace chemical detection,[3]
2. Chemical/biological sensors and mitigation of threats,
3. Millimeter wave imaging for explosives detection, and
4. Data fusion and integration for airport terminals.

By mutual agreement between the committee and the sponsor, the broad focus on "transportation security" in the statement of task was narrowed to the threat of chemical and biological attacks on the U.S. air transportation system.

The committee approached its charge by focusing on two attack settings: air terminals and aircraft. Of all the different transportation environments, the air transportation environment is perhaps the best controlled, with its checkpoints, orderly passenger flows, controlled access areas, relatively clean air, and so on. Therefore, it is likely to be the most favorable transportation environment for the application of defensive measures and technologies against terrorist attacks. Although the defensive measures and technologies discussed here may not have application to all transportation modes (e.g., containerized ships, bridges, highway tunnels), the committee believes that the air transportation security arena provides a relatively well controlled testbed for gaining experience with defensive strategies that could be adapted to other transportation spaces, such as high-value buildings, bus terminals, train stations, and cruise ships, with appropriate modifications.

As suggested by the wording of the topic of this report in the list above, this study is concerned not only with technologies for detecting the presence of chemical or biological threat agents in the air transportation context, but also with the mitigation of the impacts of their potential release. Given the very large number of technologies that are currently being investigated—both for the detection of chemical and biological agents and for the mitigation of the impact of attacks involving these agents—it was not feasible for the committee to evaluate each technology in detail. Rather, the committee chose to take a higher-level view, focusing on options for defensive strategies, as well as on the role that TSA might play in implementing these strategies. Thus, this report contains neither in-depth technical analyses nor cost-benefit analyses of specific detection systems; instead, it explores defensive strategies and options to inform the choices available to policy makers.

SCOPE OF THE REPORT

One can imagine a very large number of scenarios for attacks on the U.S. air transportation system with chemical/biological agents. This report focuses on the dispersal of threat agents in air, either in airport terminals and their boarding areas or in aircraft, as illustrated in Figure 1-1. Two kinds of agent releases are considered: point releases of agent into open spaces and releases of agent into the inlets of terminal or aircraft heating, ventilation, and air conditioning (HVAC) systems.

Chapter 2 discusses the threat posed by chemical and biological agents to the air transportation system and describes a range of attack scenarios that should be considered by government and private-sector planners. Concepts for defense against chemical/biological attacks—including those that depend on the detection of an attack before action is taken and those that do not—are explored in Chapter 3. Finally, Chapter 4 presents the committee's findings and recommendations regarding the role that TSA should play in the defense of air transportation spaces against chemical/biological attack.

[3]National Research Council, *Opportunities to Improve Airport Passenger Screening with Mass Spectrometry,* Washington, D.C.: The National Academies Press, 2004.

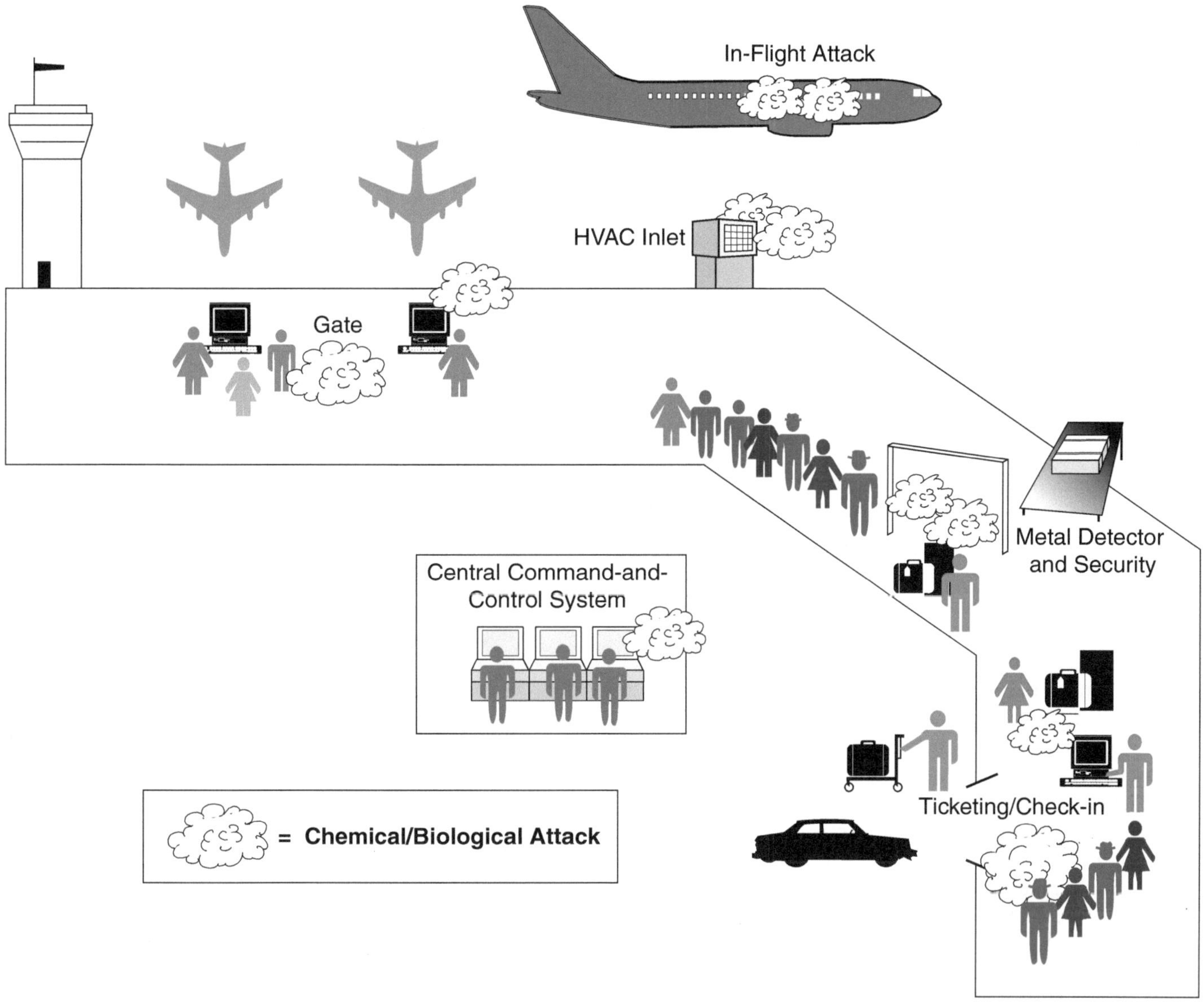

FIGURE 1-1 Generic airport diagram showing various airport spaces and some likely sites for chemical/biological attacks.

2

The Chemical/Biological Threat to Air Transportation

The focus of the antiterrorist efforts of the U.S. air transportation system to date has been on the detection of concealed arms or explosives; essentially no capability exists to detect chemical or biological warfare agents effectively and affordably or to mitigate the impact of a terrorist attack involving these agents. Thus, a terrorist runs little risk of being caught or discovered before perpetrating an attack, and the number of people exposed to the agent would depend only on how effectively the perpetrator could disseminate it.

This chapter describes examples of the chemical/biological threat agents that might be used in a terrorist attack on the U.S. air transportation system, as well as some key physical, chemical, and biological characteristics of these agents that would affect the number of people exposed to such an attack. Some plausible scenarios for the release of these agents into the air transportation environment are also discussed.

CHEMICAL/BIOLOGICAL THREAT AGENTS

Many types of threat agents might be used in an attack on the air transportation system. Each has its own set of physical, chemical, and biological characteristics, which would determine how lethal and widely dispersed the effects would be. Four different categories of threat agents can be distinguished:[1]

- *Fast-acting chemical agents.* Individuals exposed to these agents begin displaying symptoms within seconds or minutes. Examples of such agents include the neurotoxic agent sarin, the choking agent chlorine, and the blood agent hydrogen cyanide.
- *Delayed-acting chemical agents and biological toxins.* With agents in this category, which includes some chemicals as well as large-molecular-weight toxins produced by certain biological organisms, exposed individuals would not begin exhibiting symptoms for hours or days. Examples of such chemicals include sulfur mustard; biological toxins include ricin and botulinum toxin.
- *Slow-acting, noncontagious biological agents.* These agents, which include viruses as well as the bacterial causative agents for anthrax and tularemia, produce no initial symptoms, but cause flu-like symptoms after a few days or weeks. Some, such as *Bacillus anthracis,* can be disseminated either in the form of spores or as vegetative cells.
- *Slow-acting, contagious biological agents.* This category of agents, which includes the virus that causes smallpox and the bacterium that causes pneumonic plague, produces no initial symptoms upon infection but typically causes flu-like symptoms after a few days or weeks. Infected individuals are usually contagious after they are symptomatic.

Table 2-1 lists examples of agents in each of these categories, along with some of their characteristics. In the longer term, biological warfare agents may also be genetically modified to further amplify their lethality, mask their identity, protect them from vaccinates, and protect them from environmental degradation, including the effects of ultraviolet (UV) irradiation, temperature, and humidity.

Fast-Acting Versus Slow-Acting Agents

One common characteristic of many chemical agents is that they tend to be relatively fast acting: that is, victims begin to exhibit symptoms of distress within seconds to minutes after exposure to the agent. This almost-immediate showing of symptoms has implications for defensive strategies based on detection systems, since the chemical agent released in an attack would reach and produce a response

[1]Susanna Gordon, Sandia National Laboratories, in her presentation to the committee at Irvine, California, February 26, 2004.

TABLE 2-1 Examples of Chemical and Biological Threat Agents of Concern

Category	Example Agents	Initial Symptoms	Time to Symptoms\
Fast-acting chemical agents	Sarin	Convulsions, paralysis	Seconds
	Phosgene	Coughing, breathing difficulty	Seconds
	Hydrogen cyanide	Convulsions, respiratory failure	Minutes
	BZ (3-quinuclidinyle benzilate)	Delirium, hallucinations	1 hour
Delayed-acting chemical agents and biological toxins	Sulfur mustard	Blistering, redness, swelling	2 to 24 hours
	Ricin toxin	Breathing difficulty, fever, nausea	6 to 8 hours
	Botulinum toxin	Descending muscle weakness/paralysis	18 to 36 hours
Slow-acting, noncontagious biological agents	*Bacillus anthracis* (anthrax)	Flu-like symptoms	<7 days
	Francisella tularensis (tularemia)	Flu-like symptoms	3 to 5 days
Slow-acting, contagious biological agents	Variola major (smallpox)	Flu-like symptoms	12 to 14 days
	Yersinia pestis (plague)	Flu-like symptoms	1 to 6 days
	Viral hemorrhagic fever (e.g., Ebola)	Flu-like symptoms, internal bleeding	2 to 21 days

SOURCE: Centers for Disease Control and Prevention, online at http://www.bt.cdc.gov/agent/. Accessed October 6, 2005.

from the detection system at about the same time that it began producing symptoms in the exposed population. Identification of the agent involved would still be valuable for forensic purposes, but detectors would not be necessary to establish the fact of the attack itself. The implications of fast-acting agents for defensive strategies are discussed in Chapter 3.

A common characteristic of biological agents is that they are slow acting: although exposure may occur rapidly, victims' symptoms may not appear for several hours to several weeks, depending on the agent. Similarly, delayed-acting chemicals and biotoxins would produce no symptoms for several hours to several days. In that amount of time, airport passengers and workers would have dispersed to a wide variety of destinations. Thus, for attacks involving slow- or delayed-acting agents, technologies for early detection become more important—a detector alarm may be the only indicator for several days that an attack has taken place.

TABLE 2-2 Toxicities of Lethal Gases

	Respiratory (LCT_{50})	Relative Toxicities
Chlorine (Cl_2)	10,000	1
Phosgene (CG)	3,000	3
Hydrogen cyanide (AC)	5,000	2
Cyanogen chloride (CK)	11,000	1
Sulfur mustard (HD)	1,500	7
Nitrogen mustard (HN-1)	1,200	8
Tabun (GA)	400	25
Sarin (GB)	100	100
Soman (GD)	70	150
EA 5365	40	250

NOTE: LCT_{50} is the lethal concentration of toxin at which 50 percent of test animals are killed, in milligrams per minute per cubic meter.

SOURCES: *Proceedings of the Tri-Service Working Conference: Defense Against Chemical Agents—Research Needs and Opportunities*, Reston, Va., November 13-15, 1980; *The Merck Index*, 9th ed., Whitehouse Station, N.J.: Merck, 1976.

Factors Affecting the Potency of an Attack

The interplay between the chemical and biological properties of the threat agent, on the one hand, and the specific attack scenario, on the other, can influence the lethality of the attack. Table 2-2 shows the relative respiratory toxicities (expressed as the lethal concentration of toxin at which 50 percent of test animals are killed, or LCT_{50}, in milligrams per minute per cubic meter) of a variety of toxic gases compared with chlorine gas, which was used as a chemical weapon in World War I. According to Table 2-2, the nerve agent sarin (GB) has a respiratory toxicity approximately 100 times that of chlorine, while sulfur mustard (HD) is about 7 times more toxic. However, the lethality of an attack with an agent depends not only on its inherent toxicity, but also on its chemical and physical characteristics—such as volatility and vapor density—which govern its dispersion in civilian spaces. Other factors affecting the lethality of an attack include the age and overall medical condition of the individuals subject to the attack.

The chemical and physical characteristics affect exposure levels, depending on the specific attack scenario. If, for example, the agent is released at ground level and victim exposure occurs by breathing the vapor while standing, the vola-

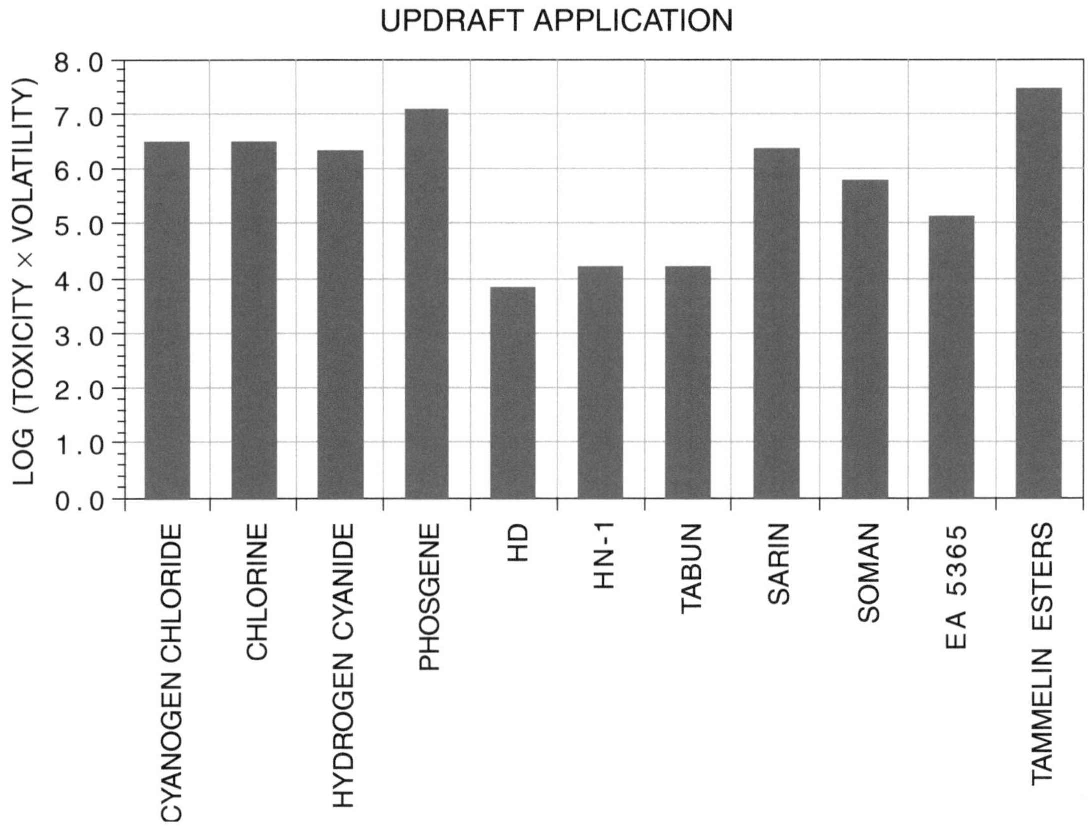

FIGURE 2-1 The relative potency of toxic gases deployed by updraft application. NOTE: These data apply primarily to diffusion-dominated dispersion of agent rather than to convection-dominated dispersion. HD, sulfur mustard; HN-1, nitrogen mustard. SOURCES: J. Enqvist et al., *Identification of Potential Organophosphorus Warfare Agents: An Approach for the Standardization of Techniques and Reference Data*, Helsinki: The Ministry for Foreign Affairs of Finland, 1979; *Handbook of Chemistry and Physics*, 63rd ed., Boca Raton, Fla.: CRC Press, 1982.

tility and density become critical factors, and higher-volatility chlorine becomes a slightly more potent agent than sarin (measured in terms of toxicity times volatility; see Figure 2-1) and much more potent than sulfur mustard, which has a relatively low volatility and high density. If, on the other hand, the agent is released above the victim and exposure occurs by breathing the vapor as it wafts down (Figure 2-2), the inherently higher toxicity of sarin and mustard gas compared with that of chlorine would become dominant in determining the potency of the attack. These considerations explain why the sarin attack on the Tokyo subway system in 1995—while horrific—did not cause more than 12 fatalities. The sarin, which has a relatively high vapor density but low volatility, was released on the floor of the subway car; had it been released from above, far more casualties would have resulted. Of course, in spaces where there are significant air currents, dispersion of the agent would occur primarily by convection rather than by diffusion, and factors such as vapor density become less important. Such air currents may occur in airport concourses where there may be external pressure differences and frequent opening and closing of doors.

In the case of biological agents, there is a range of possible delivery methods that may be used by terrorists (e.g., contamination of the water or food supply, spreading of the agent on surfaces that are touched frequently, and so on). The most effective method for infecting a large number of people in a short time, however, is likely to be that of releasing the agent into the air in the form of aerosol particles.

AIR TRANSPORTATION SPACES

In developing strategies for defending the U.S. air transportation system from chemical/biological attacks, it is important to understand the characteristics of the spaces and their human occupancy patterns. As examples, the committee considers two very different kinds of spaces: the airport terminal and the aircraft itself. Gaining an understanding of the physical configuration of these spaces, as well as entry and exit points and passenger flows, is important in deter-

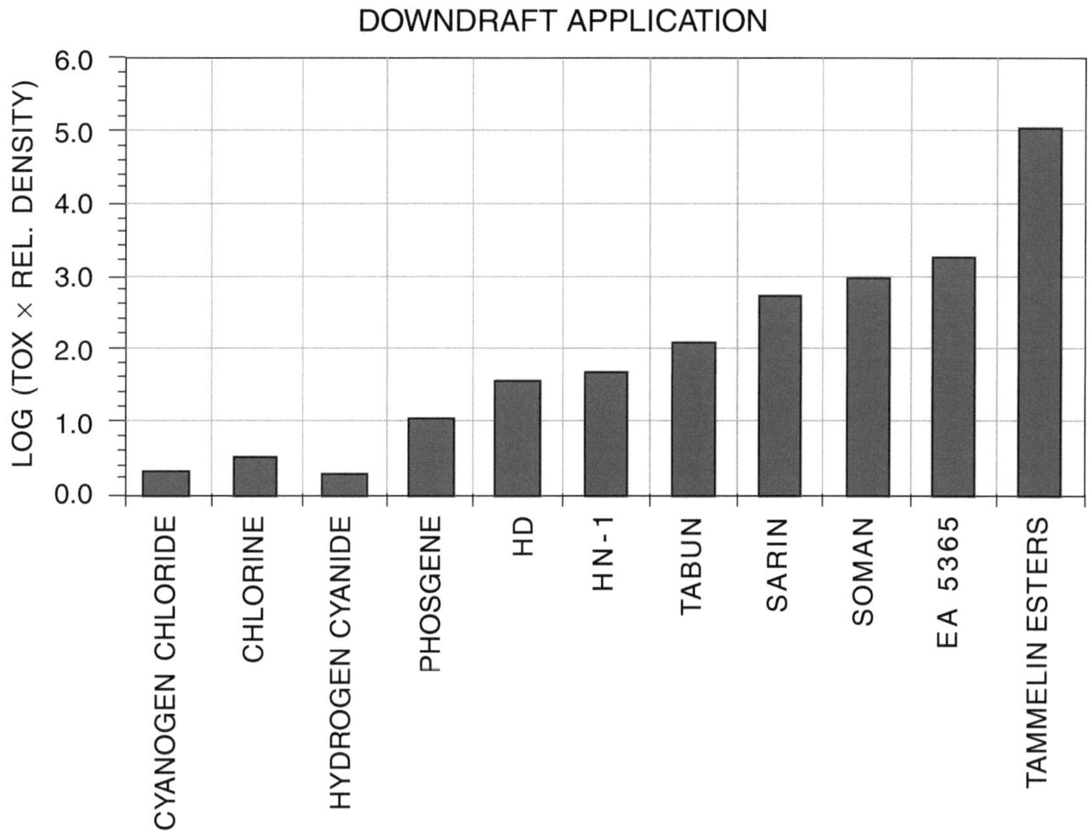

FIGURE 2-2 The relative potency of toxic gases deployed by downdraft application. NOTE: These data apply primarily to diffusion-dominated dispersion of agent rather than to convection-dominated dispersion. HD, sulfur mustard; HN-1, nitrogen mustard. SOURCES: J. Enqvist et al., *Identification of Potential Organophosphorus Warfare Agents: An Approach for the Standardization of Techniques and Reference Data*, Helsinki: The Ministry for Foreign Affairs of Finland, 1979; *Handbook of Chemistry and Physics*, 63rd ed., Boca Raton, Fla.: CRC Press, 1982.

mining vulnerabilities and potential choke points at which large numbers of people might gather and be exposed to attacks. Since the committee's focus is on attacks involving releases of agents into the air, understanding the airflow patterns in these spaces is particularly important. By empirically studying and modeling the occupancy patterns, physical characteristics, and airflow patterns in these spaces, one can begin to understand how chemical/biological threat agents might be dispersed and what strategies might be most appropriate for defending against them. The discussion below is intended to identify some of the factors that may be important in the assembly of such models.

Airport Terminals

Airport terminals are typically large, open spaces with relatively uniform physical configurations that include, for example, ticketing/check-in areas, baggage claim areas, security checkpoints, concessions, restrooms, and departure gates. These large spaces require heating, ventilation, and air conditioning (HVAC) systems to maintain acceptable air quality. Some areas are open to the general public, and others are restricted to passengers, employees, and/or security personnel. Access to the various spaces is less well controlled in other transportation venues such as bus, railway, and shipping terminals, presumably because there has been no history of attacks against such facilities in the United States.

Terminals generally accommodate the large numbers of the traveling public that move through them with residence times of about 1 to 2 hours. There are also large numbers of visitors who are not traveling but are dropping off travelers at check-in areas or waiting to meet travelers in the baggage claim areas. Their stay at the facility would typically be at least 30 minutes, although such assumptions should be checked against actual data. In addition, there are a significant number of airline, concessions, ground transportation, and security personnel working within airport terminals around the clock. In passenger ticketing/check-in areas, there are numerous entry and exit points. Data and models are needed for flow behavior of people both during normal

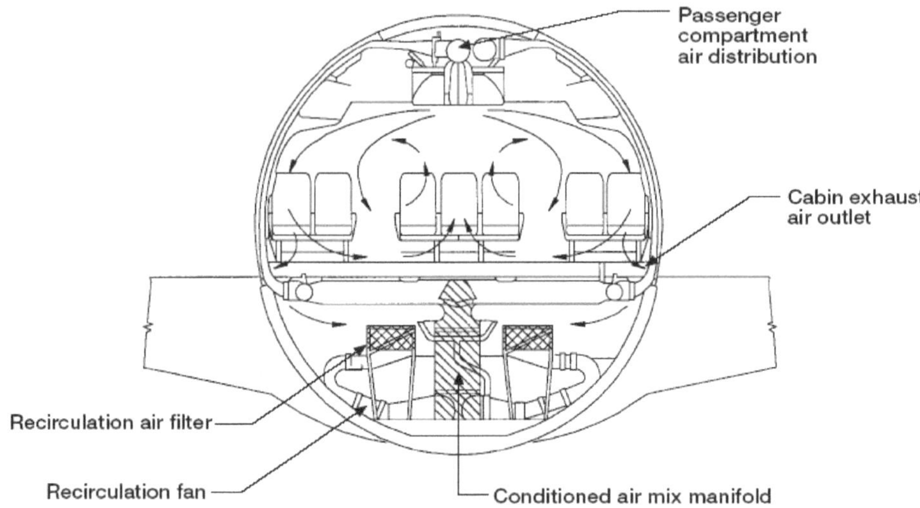

FIGURE 2-3 Airflow patterns in a typical passenger aircraft. SOURCE: Available online at http://www.boeing.com/commercial/cabinair/ecs.pdf. Accessed October 7, 2005.

airport operations and after being alerted to a potential hazard.

Most passengers are carrying at least one bag, if not more, and a very large number of checked bags are passing through the facility from check-in areas to aircraft. There is a constant movement of materials and supplies throughout all areas of the facility, and large amounts of cargo and shipping containers are also moved through on their way to the aircraft. From the point of view of a terrorist, these relatively invariant characteristics of airport terminals may suggest logical points of attack. Similarly, they can provide the basis for a rational design of a defense against such an attack.

Aircraft

The aircraft itself comprises space very different from that of the terminal. The cabin features a relatively small, confined space with a very high density of passengers, crew, and carry-on bags. The minimum passenger residence time on an aircraft is about 1 hour, with maximum times stretching to 14 hours for very long distance flights. Well-publicized penalties for deviant passenger behavior and for failure to obey crew instructions have conditioned passengers to behave in a more compliant manner than can be expected in terminals. Airflow is also better controlled in an aircraft.

Virtually all aircraft have the same basic physical configuration. The Environmental Control System (ECS) is crucial for maintaining air quality during a flight, and the vast majority of aircraft have similar localized airflow patterns (Figure 2-3). During a flight on a typical airliner, 50 percent of outside air is mixed with 50 percent filtered, recirculated air, with complete exchange of the cabin air volume every 2 to 3 minutes.[2] Special consideration is given to air supplied to the cockpit.

[2]Information is available online at http://www.boeing.com/commercial/cabinair/. Accessed October 5, 2005.

Although there are few access points to an aircraft before a flight and although passenger access is carefully controlled, a significant number of airport personnel have access to the aircraft between flights. These include baggage handlers, cleaners, food service personnel, maintenance personnel, and refuelers. In addition, while the aircraft is on the ground, it is connected to an external HVAC system. These various factors suggest that aircraft face a significant vulnerability to chemical/biological attacks while they are on the ground.

ATTACK SCENARIOS

The committee was not given specific attack scenarios to consider in this study, either in terms of the spaces attacked, the agents involved, or the manner of agent release. Accordingly, the discussion below is qualitative, intended to highlight some of the factors that need to be considered in forming appropriate defensive strategies against such attacks. As noted above, only an air release of agent is considered here.[3]

Point Release Versus Attack on the Heating, Ventilation, and Air Conditioning System

In a point release attack, the agent would be released in a plume from a single point (or perhaps several discrete points simultaneously). Individuals near the point of release would be exposed to agent at high levels, whereas those farther away would be exposed at lower doses. Initially, the spread of agent would be confined to the space in which it was

[3]Examples of potential chemical attack scenarios are identified in a Federal Aviation Administration (FAA)-funded study undertaken at Johns Hopkins University: *Chemical Sensing and Mitigation Options for Commercial Airliners*, Final Report, STD-01-189, Laurel, Md.: Johns Hopkins University Applied Physics Laboratory, July 2001.

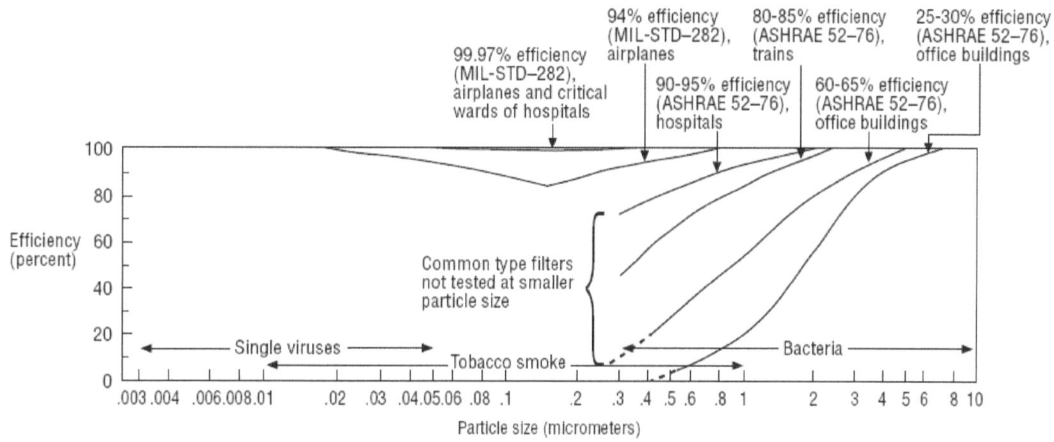

FIGURE 2-4 Filter removal efficiencies for particles of various sizes. NOTE: In an attack with a large quantity of aerosolized agent, the removal efficiencies shown here might not be high enough to prevent widespread exposure and symptoms, particularly with highly infectious agents. MIL-STD: Military Standard; ASHRAE: American Society of Heating, Refrigeration, and Air Conditioning Engineers. SOURCE: Available online at http://www.boeing.com/commercial/cabinair/ecs.pdf. Accessed October 7, 2005.

originally released; subsequently, it might spread considerably via air drift down corridors and from level to level through mezzanines and stairwells. If HVAC systems continued to operate, the agent would be drawn into the ductwork and spread to connected rooms or spaces, albeit with considerable dilution.

If the agent were released directly into the inlet of an HVAC system that had no associated air treatment technologies, it would be pumped through the ductwork into all of the connected spaces, creating the potential for simultaneous, widespread exposures to relatively high concentrations of agent. Although this scenario is of particular concern owing to the potential for mass casualties, the confined nature of an HVAC system offers a number of possibilities for defense, as discussed in Chapter 3.

Aerosol particles in the 1- to 10-micrometer (μm) size range are removed from the air with fairly high efficiency (>50 percent) by common building HVAC air filters, and with very high efficiency (>99.97 percent) by the high-efficiency particulate air (HEPA) filters in the ECS of a modern airliner (Figure 2-4).[4] Nevertheless, in an attack with a large quantity of aerosolized agent, these removal efficiencies might not be high enough to prevent widespread exposure and symptoms, particularly with highly infectious agents. Chemical agents are typically small organic molecules (not associated with particles) that would not be removed by common air-filtration systems. Air can be cleansed of organic chemical contaminants by passing it through a bed of highly adsorbent material such as activated carbon with appropriate additives, or other sorbents, and/or through an active (e.g., plasma) sterilization chamber.

Attacks Involving Fast- Versus Slow-Acting Agents

Some of the characteristics of fast- and slow-acting agents have been discussed above. An attack on the air transportation system with a fast-acting (chemical) agent would likely occur in an area in which large numbers of people were gathered, either in a terminal or in an aircraft. The fact of the attack would quickly become obvious as victims began to collapse or exhibit other symptoms of distress. It would be important for the authorities to recognize quickly that an attack had occurred in order to facilitate evacuation, get medical help for the victims, and limit the access of nonessential personnel to the contaminated area. If the attack occurred in an aircraft passenger cabin during a flight, the aircraft might be brought down (or taken over by terrorists) if the pilots became incapacitated. Similarly, attacks on critical nodes within an airport terminal (control rooms, emergency-response centers, and so on) could incapacitate key decision makers or deny authorities the use of these spaces, so as to prevent an effective response.

[4]These efficiencies assume proper, leak-free installation. Filters are often improperly installed and sometimes missing. Reliance on filtration requires a quality-assurance program to ensure that filters are in place and functioning.

In contrast, in the absence of an effective detection or air-treatment system, an attack involving a slow-acting agent might go unrecognized for days, until the exposed victims began exhibiting symptoms of disease. Since the incubation periods for the appearance of symptoms of illness caused by slow-acting agents are typically long compared with the residence time of travelers in an airport terminal or aircraft, victims would be geographically dispersed by the time symptoms had appeared, and it might be difficult to locate them. If the disease were communicable, it could be spread by infected passengers to far-flung parts of the world in a very short time. An intentionally infected passenger (i.e., a suicide terrorist) traveling on a long flight could be one efficient means of infecting other passengers with a slow-acting biological agent. Unlike the situation created by a fast-acting agent, however, the problems caused by the release of a slow-acting agent in flight would not be an effective way of bringing down an aircraft. In the specialized case of very large releases of anthrax spores, the attacked aircraft could provide a means of infecting passengers over the course of multiple flights owing to the high survival capability of spore-forming bacteria.

Quantity and Rate of Release of Agent

The quantity of agent used in an attack and its rate of release are also factors that a terrorist, and thus a defender, must consider. In manufacturing, transporting, or preparing for the release of a large quantity of agent, the terrorist would risk being discovered before the attack could be perpetrated. Similarly, if a slow-acting agent were released at a high rate, there would be a higher probability that the attack would be observed or would cause a detector (if present) to alarm, since the ambient concentration would likely be well above the detector threshold. By comparison, a slow release rate ("trickle attack") and a highly infectious agent might produce ambient agent levels that are below the threshold of available detection systems, yet sufficient to infect exposed individuals. This would be balanced against the increased time required to carry out the attack, with the associated increased risk of discovery.

3

Defensive Strategies

This chapter discusses two kinds of defensive strategies for protecting U.S. air transportation spaces from chemical/biological attacks: one type is based on detecting an attack through a technological sensor-based detection system and then reacting in an appropriate way; the other type involves taking actions that can ameliorate or help prevent an attack without reliance on a detection event. One example of the latter approach would be continuously cleaning the air to remove contaminants. These two strategies are not mutually exclusive; indeed, they can be complementary for certain attack scenarios.

DETECTION-BASED STRATEGIES

In a defensive strategy that is based on the detection of a chemical/biological agent in order to initiate a response, the time required for authorities to respond to an attack has three components: the inherent response time of the detection system, the time required to verify the validity of a detector alarm, and the time required to decide on what action to take in response to the alarm. These three elements are discussed in more detail below.

Response Time of the Detection System

The detection of harmful substances in air requires time. Three kinds of detection schemes are discussed here: (1) continuous chemical sensors (Figure 3-1) and (2) discontinuous chemical-detection systems, both of which might be suitable for the detection of both fast- and delayed-acting chemical agents, and (3) biosensing systems (see Figure 3-2), which would typically be used to detect and/or identify biological (slow-acting) agents.

The signal from continuous chemical sensors is continuous in time. It follows changes in the concentration of the analyte up and down. The signal often originates from the interaction of the analyte with a chemically selective layer on the sensor.[1] This interaction can occur either in the bulk of the layer or at its surface. The signal is then amplified by the transducer using one of four basic types of amplification mechanisms—thermal, mass, electrochemical, or optical—listed in Figure 3-1. The continuous signal typically enables the chemical sensor to respond quickly to large changes in the concentration of the target analyte, which would occur, for example, with a nearby release of chemical agents.

Discontinuous chemical-detection systems do not provide a signal that is continuous in time, but rather cycle rapidly through a series of phases such as sample collection, preconcentration, separation, and detection in such a way that the overall system is capable of providing a detection report every minute or so. Examples of such systems include ion mobility spectrometers, mass spectrometers, and chromatography-based systems. Many technologies are possible candidates for each of the different phases.[2]

The distinction between "detection" and "identification" is important, since it may affect the overall response time and options. A *detection* occurs when a chosen parameter exceeds its threshold value. The detection may be nonspecific—that is, it registers the occurrence of an anomaly but does not necessarily indicate the presence of a particular threat substance. By contrast, *identification* establishes the identity of the threat substances in a given set. Nonspecific detection systems may have a relatively rapid response time compared with that of specific identification systems, but the former typically provide a lower confidence level that a threat substance is in fact present. In some cases, an alarm from a rapid but nonspecific detection system may be used

---

[1]Sensors that operate on the basis of interactive chemical surfaces are chosen for discussion here because they are likely candidates for the detection of chemical agents. However, many other sensor types are possible.

[2]Figure 4-2 in the next chapter offers a partial list of technologies being investigated for various stages of chemical/biological agent detection systems.

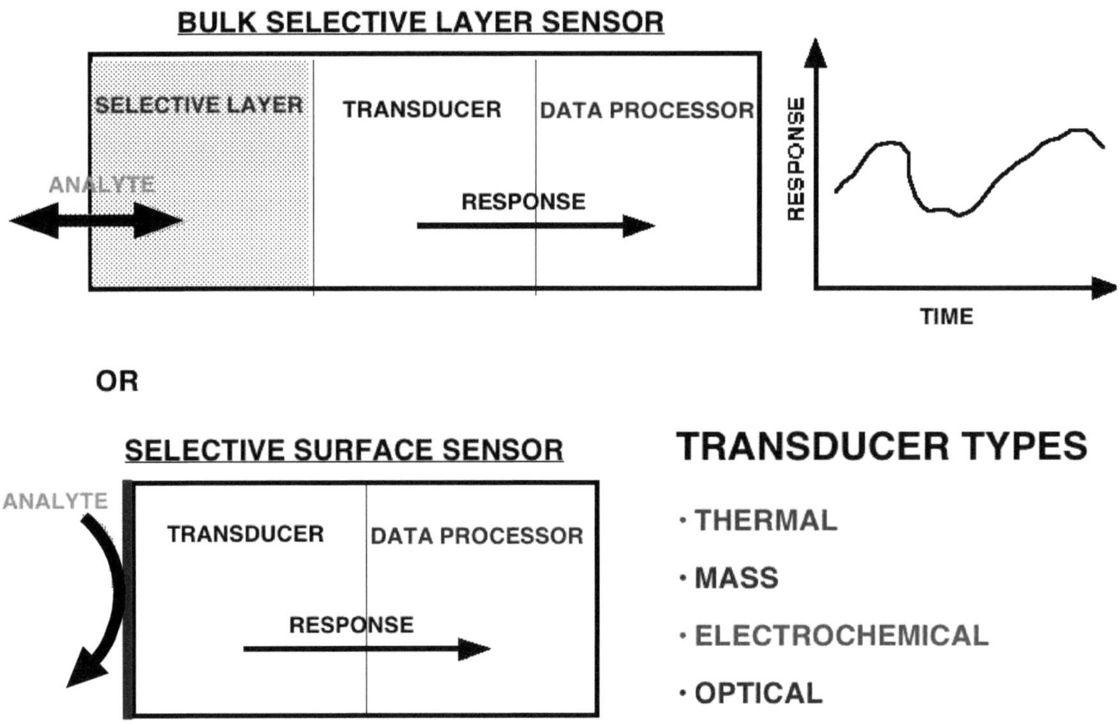

FIGURE 3-1 Operational schematic of continuous chemical sensors.

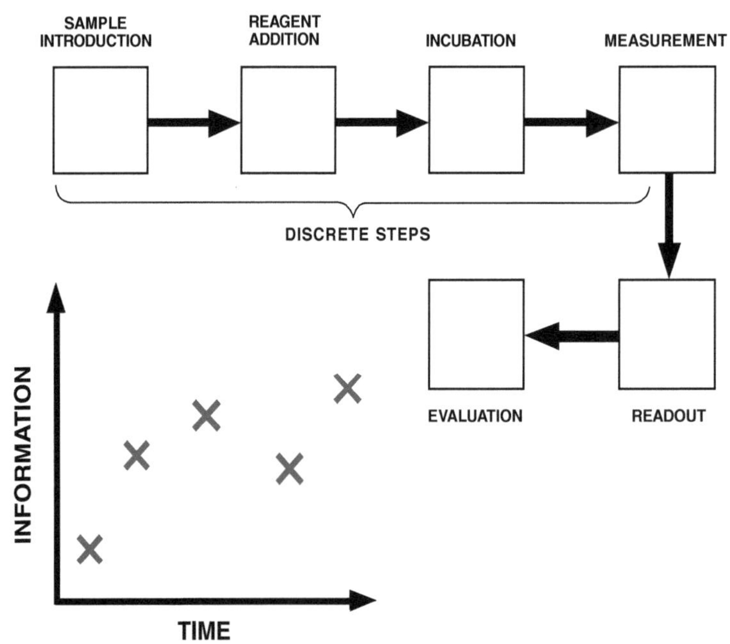

FIGURE 3-2 Operational schematic of discontinuous biosensing system (assay).

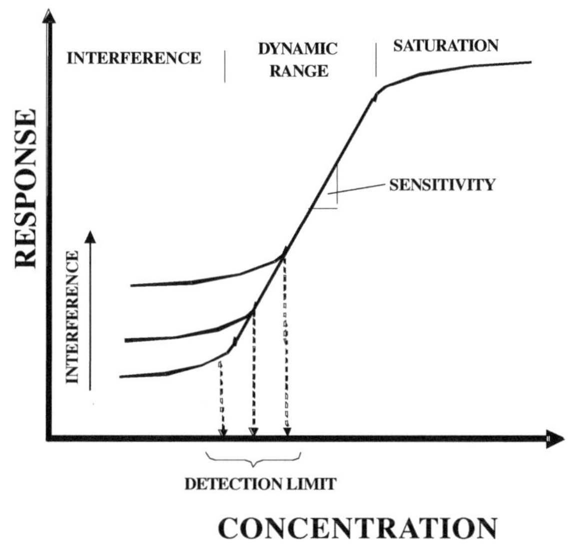

FIGURE 3-3 Key characteristics of sensor systems (see discussion in text).

to initiate "low-regret" responses (those that could provide some protection to potentially exposed people without causing too much disruption—e.g., shutting down a heating, ventilation, and air conditioning [HVAC] system) or to trigger an analysis by a more specific, but slower, identification system.

The response curves of all analytical methods, including continuous sensors and discrete assays, have important common characteristics, shown in Figure 3-3. The range of concentrations in which the sensor responds is called the dynamic range. It is bounded on its upper end by the saturation limit and on its lower end by the detection limit. Increasing concentrations of interfering compounds shift the detection limit to higher concentrations, thus reducing the dynamic range. Therefore, the detection limit always depends on the chemical complexity of the sample. The sensitivity is the slope of the response curve in the dynamic range.

As with discontinuous chemical-detection systems, the information derived from a biosensing system or assay is discontinuous in time. As noted above, the discontinuous chemical detector may be capable of cycling through its stages and providing a report every minute or so, whereas an assay typically takes some hours to complete. The assay consists of two or more discrete steps, such as sample introduction, addition of reagents, incubation with reagents, measurement of signal, and so on, as shown in Figure 3-2.[3] Considerable time is generally required *before* the steps shown in Figure 3-2 to acquire the sample and prepare it for the assay (e.g., concentration, separation from background contaminants, lysing of cells to release the target moiety, and so on). The acquisition of the sample always determines time $t = 0$ for the sequence. In other words, even if a biological agent release occurs in the vicinity of the detection system at time t, the analysis sequence does not begin until the next sample acquisition time.

Typical times required to complete the detection steps for chemical and biological agents are shown on the left-hand side of Figure 3-4. In the case of chemicals, the total time required for sampling, measurement, and evaluation is typically less than 1 minute. In the case of biological agents, the assay typically takes longer than 1 hour to perform. For example, in a typical assay involving the binding of target DNA strands to complementary strands on a sensor surface, the incubation time to achieve a measurable signal is about 1 hour. In the case of both chemicals and biological agents, the quality of the analysis is a function of agent type and concentration, as well as the complexity of the environment in which it is detected.

In general, there is a trade-off between the time required to obtain analytical results and the specificity of the information desired: for example, it may take somewhat less time to determine that an unusually high level of biological particles is present in the air (nonspecific detection) and considerably longer to identify the specific biological organisms associated with those particles.[4] Detection systems that provide continuous monitoring of airborne organic-based particles in the respirable 1 to 10 μm size range are currently available via laser-based technologies employing Mie scattering and ultraviolet (UV) fluorescence techniques.[5] These methods are significantly less sensitive and specific[6] than the biological assays discussed above and would have to be validated by rigorous field tests to ensure that they have an acceptably low false-alarm rate; however, in the future they could potentially detect very large attacks with particle counts much higher than the background, or serve as a real-time "trigger" for the initiation of a more specific detection technology. Given the potentially lengthy period that may be

[3]The lengthy assay described here may well provide specific information about the identity of the components of the biological sample. More rapid—but less specific—information may be obtained from other technologies, such as the bioaerosol detectors discussed below.

[4]National Research Council, *Sensor Systems for Biological Agent Attacks: Protecting Buildings and Military Bases*, Washington, D.C.: The National Academies Press, 2005.

[5]National Research Council, *Sensor Systems for Biological Agent Attacks: Protecting Buildings and Military Bases*, Washington, D.C.: The National Academies Press, 2005.

[6]More chemical-specific bioaerosol detectors are also being explored. See, for example, D.P. Fergenson, M.E. Pitesky, H.J. Tobias, P.T. Steele, G.A. Czerwieniec, S.C. Russell, C.B. LeBrilla, J.M. Horn, K.R. Coffee, A. Srivastava, S.P. Pillai, M-T.P. Shih, H.L. Hall, A.J. Ramponi, J.T. Chang, R.G. Langlois, P.L. Estacio, R.T. Hadley, M. Frank, and E.E. Gard, "Reagentless Detection and Classification of Individual Bioaerosol Particles in Seconds," Anal. Chem., Vol. 76, pp. 373-378, 2004.

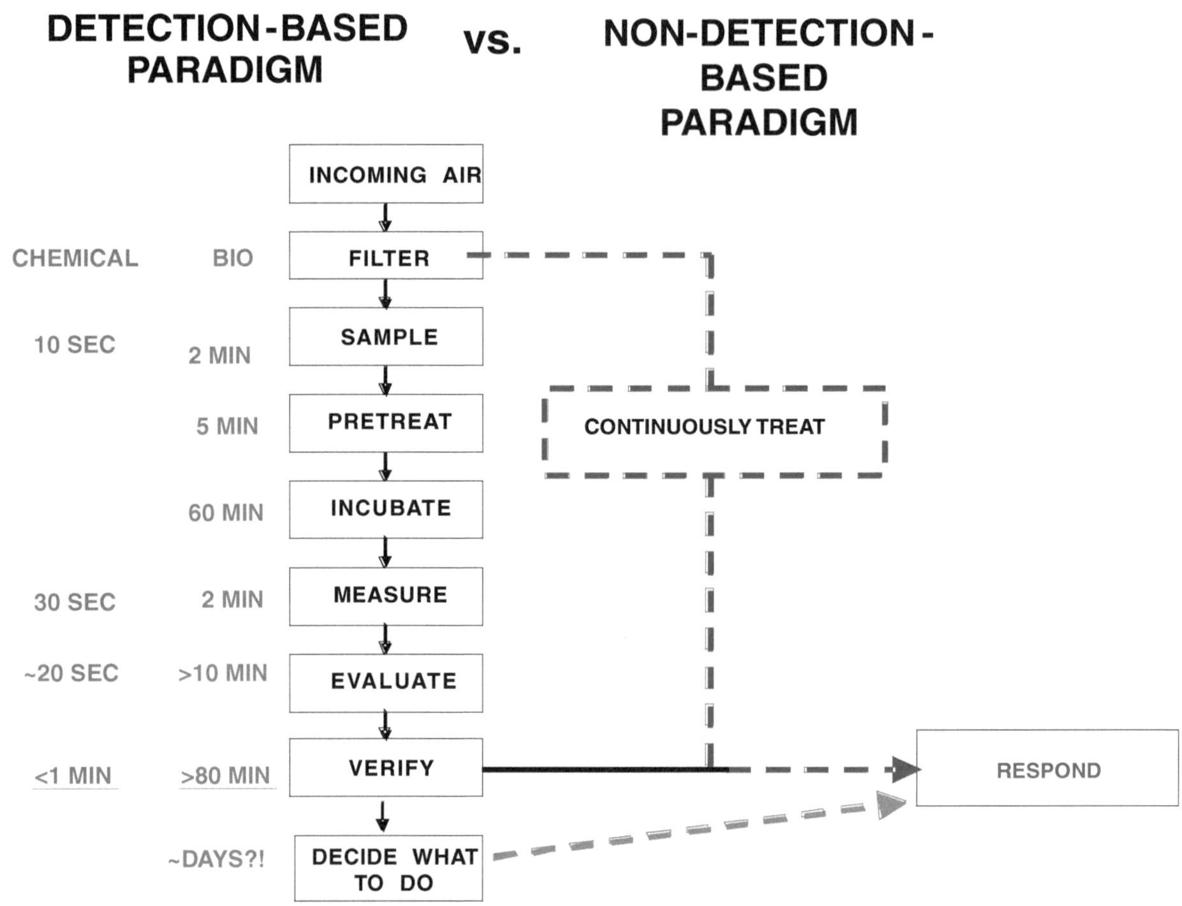

FIGURE 3-4 Typical detection times for chemical and biological agents (left-hand side). A strategy based on continuous air treatment (dashed lines) bypasses many time-consuming steps required in a chemical/biological agent detector-based strategy, including the response decision step at the end. NOTE: While continuous air treatment (the non-detection-based paradigm) does not eliminate exposure of individuals in the vicinity of a chemical/biological agent release, it does begin immediately to mitigate the consequences of an attack, avoiding the often-lengthy delays for a response associated with the detection-based paradigm.

required to fully identify the specific organisms that may have caused a detector to alarm, it may be desirable to initiate a response before the final identification is completed.

Time to Verify Alarm Validity

All detection systems feature a trade-off between the probability of detection (POD) of the target substance and the probability of false (positive) alarms (PFA). POD refers to the probability that the instrument will detect a threat material that is present; PFA refers to the probability that the instrument will alarm when a threat material is not present at a given threshold level. The overall concentration of the target substance affects this trade-off: higher concentrations are easier to detect, resulting in performance closer to the optimum operating point (perfect detection with zero false alarms). In addition, where data are accumulated over time, one can increase POD and decrease PFA by increasing the accumulation time.

Depending on the performance of the detection system technology (that is, on the POD and PFA), one might have greater or less confidence that an alarm represented a real chemical/biological attack, and if PFA were significant it would be necessary to have an independent means (e.g., a separate detection technology) of verifying the validity of the alarm. This process would take additional time—the alarm resolution time. In some cases, it might be possible to initiate certain low-regret responses while an alarm was being resolved.

The trade-off between POD and PFA is affected by the alarm threshold setting of the instrument; a low alarm threshold results in a higher POD but also more frequent false alarms, whereas a higher threshold results in a lower POD as well as a lower PFA. A higher threshold increases the rate of false negatives—that is, the instrument fails to alarm when the threat material is present. By combining two orthogonal detection technologies, one can lower the detection threshold and the false-alarm rate achievable with a single technology, although at a higher cost.

One reason for false alarms from detection systems is the presence of interfering molecules or organisms from the background environment that may be present in the sample. These may be chemically or biologically similar to the target threat agents, causing a similar response in the detector. Thus, the specificity of the detection system (i.e., its ability to distinguish the target analyte from the background) is a critical factor determining its performance. Although chemical threat agents tend to be quite distinct from most background molecules likely to be encountered in the airport environment, the same may not be true of biological agents. The conditions in an airport terminal, in which large numbers of people are coming and going, removing coats, coughing, and so on, are likely to produce a significant and fluctuating background of biological aerosol particles that could mimic the fluctuations likely to be seen in an attack with biological agents and therefore create false alarms. In the case of some threat agents (e.g., anthrax or plague), there may also be small natural concentrations in the environment that could trigger false alarms. In order to set detection thresholds appropriately and to minimize false alarms, it will be important to characterize the background levels and fluctuations of various kinds of relevant bioaerosol particles over time and in various airport locations.

Time Required for Deciding How to Respond

Once a chemical/biological detector has alarmed, authorities must make decisions about how to respond. One immediate action is to try to determine the validity of the alarm, as discussed above. In general, the level of response should be commensurate with the level of confidence that the alarm reflects a real terrorist attack. In the case of an attack with slow-acting agents, the alarm may be the only indication that an attack has taken place. Thus, if the detection system has a relatively high PFA, or if the identification of the organisms causing the alarm will require an extended period, an appropriate initial response may be to initiate low-regret actions such as shutting down the HVAC system or increasing the pressure in adjacent air spaces, rather than immediately notifying the potentially exposed individuals that they need to seek medical attention. However, if the detection system has a very low PFA, more extreme responses may be appropriate. The POD/PFA trade-off can be used to evaluate the effects of the various alarm settings and response policies, noting again that there is a trade-off between decision quality (high POD, low PFA) and response time.

To minimize the time needed to make a decision on the response to choose in a detection-based defensive strategy, it is necessary to have contingency plans in place for responding appropriately to the alarm situations likely to be encountered. These plans should include an array of options of graduated intensity keyed to the quality of information available. They should include emergency changes to the operation of the HVAC system, evacuation of potentially exposed individuals, isolation of affected terminal areas and passengers in order to limit additional exposures, notification of passengers and workers potentially exposed who may have left the area, provision of supplies for early medical treatment, and decontamination of affected areas to facilitate timely reopening of the facility and to minimize the economic impact of an attack. Response time will be reduced if the roles and responsibilities of all the various decision-making authorities (those in charge of airport operations, security, fire prevention and control, health and safety, environmental protection, and so on) are clearly defined and coordinated, and appropriate plan documents, required approvals (e.g., for decontamination plans), and training are in place ahead of time.[7]

Of equal importance is that decision makers have a well-designed visual display of the information needed to make the appropriate decision and that they are well practiced in making decisions under time urgency. If the political and economic consequences of a course of action are great, the decision time for response is likely to be longer. There has been little research on these important aspects of human decision making in the security context, although much relevant research is available from comparable domains, such as operating rooms and fire-control centers.

Improved Visual Surveillance

As discussed above, in an attack involving the use of a fast-acting chemical/biological agent, it is likely that released agent would begin producing symptoms in the exposed population before or at about the same time that the agent reached any deployed detector. Therefore, the fastest "detector" of this type of attack may be the visual observation that individuals in the terminal or aircraft are collapsing or behaving in an unusual manner. One option for improving the capacity to recognize such attacks rapidly would be to deploy enough surveillance cameras to observe the spaces where large numbers of people gather and to feed the output back to a central monitoring point. Unlike a technological detector, which is only capable of responding to a limited number of toxic chemicals that have been anticipated and whose signatures have been placed in a reference library, the surveillance camera is a "functional detector" that can be expected to "see" the effects of all fast-acting toxic chemicals that are present in sufficient concentration to cause symptoms.

Given the large amount of data generated by surveillance cameras and the infrequency of attacks, human monitors would require a technological alert system, and the overall response time to a possible attack might well be reduced if

[7] *Summary of the 2003 San Francisco International Airport Bio-Defense Preparation Exercise*, Sandia Report SAND2004-2225, Albuquerque, N.Mex.: Sandia National Laboratories, May 2004.

human monitors were provided with technological backup. Software programs could be developed that could be trained to recognize crowd behavior patterns that would be characteristic of an attack with a fast-acting chemical/biological agent, and these could provide a rapid, continuous method of monitoring the surveillance data.[8] The issue will be the optimum allocation of function between humans and algorithms to maximize POD while minimizing PFA. Neither humans nor algorithms alone are completely effective for these purposes; hybrid systems typically produce better performance.

Critique of Detection-Based Defensive Strategies

As outlined above, a critical parameter determining the value of a detection-based strategy for defense against chemical/biological attacks is response time. In an attack involving a fast-acting agent, the agent would reach the detector and produce a response in about the same amount of time that it took to begin producing symptoms in the exposed population. If a chemical-detector system were reliable, were sensitive to most possible attack agents, and had an acceptably low false-alarm rate, such an alarm could have value in confirming the fact of an attack, helping to pinpoint its location, or alerting authorities to a possible release of agent in unoccupied areas of a facility. Furthermore, if the detector could identify the agent used unambiguously, this information could help in formulating an appropriate response and speeding up the administration of antidotes and subsequent medical treatments. Such an early-warning detector might be particularly useful in some scenarios, such as the release of agent in an unoccupied area that could migrate to occupied areas, or a release into air intakes.

The value of a detection-based strategy in responding to an attack involving a slow-acting agent depends on the response time. If the detection can be made within about a minute of the initiation of such an attack, the spread of the agent may be limited to the area in the vicinity of the release, and it may be possible to warn and evacuate individuals who are farther away, thus preventing their exposure. If the detection can be made within approximately 1 hour (a typical passenger residence time in an air terminal), it may be possible to notify the potentially exposed population before people leave the area and isolate the affected area so as to limit new exposures. Provision needs to be made for safe-handling areas and procedures for any sources of hazard. If the detection of slow-acting agent can be made within several hours, it may be possible to alert potentially exposed populations through news broadcasts and other mass-media outlets to seek medical treatment or to divert, land, and quarantine affected airplanes. Even if a detection is not made for several days, an identification of the specific organisms involved and analysis of any factors that make them unique can aid the medical treatment of victims, the restoration of affected areas, and the forensic investigation to find the perpetrators.[9]

It is likely that with continued investment in research and development, it will be possible in the future to reduce the detection time for biological agent attacks below 1 hour, while maintaining or increasing the POD.[10] A faster response time with high POD would increase the benefits of detection systems and the effectiveness of detection-based strategies.

The feasibility of detection-based defensive strategies depends on the performance and cost of detection systems. Some of the factors that determine performance have been discussed above (e.g., POD and PFA, sampling frequency, assay analysis time). Others factors include the detection limit (the smallest amount detectable, always a function of the chemical or biological specificity); the detector sensitivity (the ability to detect small changes in the target concentration); the chemical specificity (the ability to separate analyte from background); and the range of agents that can be simultaneously detected. Further, a well-designed operator interface and training are needed to help the operator establish an appropriate level of trust in the system. Cost factors include the initial cost of the instrumentation as well as the recurring operating costs for maintenance, calibration, replacement of spent reagents, regeneration of the sensor surfaces, and other assay costs, including training and labor costs.

A successful detection system would have to be capable of detecting a large palette of chemical/biological agents simultaneously. This would likely require an array of sensor elements that would respond in a unique way to different agents. Nevertheless, the system would only be capable of recognizing agent signatures that had been anticipated and included in a reference "library." This problem, together with the fact that there are thousands of toxic chemicals that could potentially be used in a terrorist attack, represents a fundamental limitation on the technological detection-based strategy. The situation is somewhat better in the case of a biological attack, since the range of agents that could be used in practice is significantly smaller. Unanticipated agents, those whose signatures had been modified by an attack perpetrator, or those deliberately embedded in complex mixtures of interfering compounds might well go undetected.

[8] See, for example, information available at http://www.vistascape.com. Accessed October 11, 2005.

[9] An additional option might be the collection of historical air samples for later analysis if an attack is suspected. However, there is a significant cost to collecting and storing samples, and these costs may well outweigh the expected benefits.

[10] National Research Council, *Sensor Systems for Biological Agent Attacks: Protecting Buildings and Military Bases*, Washington, D.C.: The National Academies Press, 2005.

The feasibility of detection-based defensive strategies also depends on how the detectors are deployed and how they are actually used. Deployment considerations include the number and placement of detectors, whether in open spaces or in HVAC ductwork. In this respect, airport terminals are likely to be more difficult to protect by this strategy than are aircraft, owing to the vastly greater air volume and necessarily greater physical spacing between detectors in terminals. To the extent that more than one type of independent detection or verification system is needed to achieve acceptable POD and PFA, the system costs are multiplied.

NON-DETECTION-BASED DEFENSIVE STRATEGIES

Defensive strategies that do not depend on the technological detection of a chemical/biological attack include steps that can be taken prior to any attack to reduce the probability of the attack or to reduce its severity, and the use of continuous air treatment to remove all contaminants. For attacks involving slow-acting agents, these strategies obviate the lengthy delays needed for sample collection, preparation, assay, and reporting (see dashed lines of Figure 3-4 and the discussion below).

Proactive Steps

Steps for preventing or deterring a chemical/biological attack might include improved security—for example, ensuring that only authorized personnel have access to the air intakes of terminal HVAC systems and the ventilation systems connected to aircraft on the ground. As noted in Chapter 2, the air intakes in terminals could be used to rapidly spread threat agents throughout a large area in any attack. More visible security personnel might also have a deterrent effect on would-be perpetrators.

Proactive steps that could help to mitigate the impact of any such attack include balancing the air-handling systems in different regions of the terminal to reduce drafts that could spread threat agents (although with thousands of people coming and going, the effectiveness and practicality of this step would have to be verified), and enabling the rapid shutdown of HVAC systems in the event of a suspected attack in order to reduce the spread of agents. Empirical studies involving the transport of released agent simulants in various transportation spaces could help to illustrate how threat agents having various physical, chemical, and biological properties would spread through the spaces; this process could help create suggestions of other proactive steps that might be taken.[11] It might also be prudent to ensure that critical spaces within the air transportation system (emergency-control rooms, control towers, and so on) have access to an independent supply of clean air and are maintained at a positive pressure with respect to their surroundings, in order to reduce the likelihood that chemical/biological agents released in surrounding publicly accessible areas might disrupt these critical nodes.

Continuous Air Treatment

The strategy of continuous air treatment would be aimed at providing "clean air" to all users of transportation spaces, both in airport terminals and aircraft. This approach would be analogous to that of municipal water-treatment programs that continuously treat water supplies so as to provide clean water to city residents. The current "gold standard" for air cleaning in hospitals and industrial clean rooms is a combination of high-efficiency particulate air (HEPA) filters to remove particles along with carbon adsorbent filters to remove organic compounds. This approach can be expensive and bulky; in addition, carbon filters have a limited capacity and so must be changed at regular intervals. Other approaches being explored include catalytic oxidation of the air stream and use of hybrid systems such as a plasma oxidation pretreatment followed by carbon filtration, in which the plasma oxidation helps to offset the limited capacity of the carbon.

Given the much smaller air volume inside an aircraft as compared with that in an airport terminal, it could be technically easier and cheaper to implement the continuous air-treatment strategy in an aircraft.[12] As discussed in Chapter 2, the air filtration system in modern airliners efficiently removes particulate matter, including aerosolized pathogens, that passes through them, although current filter systems would not provide protection against fast-acting chemical agents.

In terminal areas, the air volumes are much greater, and typical HVAC filtration systems do not remove aerosol particles from the air as efficiently as do aircraft Environmental Control Systems (see Chapter 2). Thus, the costs and benefits of various enhanced filtration and air-cleaning strategies would have to be carefully assessed. An ancillary benefit to be considered would be the reduction of the transmission of common ills such as cold and flu viruses (or more serious viruses, such as the severe acute respiratory syndrome [SARS] virus) among airport patrons.

Critique of the Non-Detection-Based Strategy

A defensive strategy against chemical/biological attacks that does not rely on a detection event to initiate a response

---

[11]See, for example, *Tracer Release Experiments at San Francisco International Airport to Improve Preparedness Against Chemical and Biological Terrorism*, Sandia Report SAND2001-8380, Albuquerque, N.Mex.: Sandia National Laboratories, June 2001.

[12]The added cost, weight, reliability, and maintenance implications would have to be weighed against the expected benefits.

has many appealing aspects. It would avoid many problems: the likely high cost of purchasing and operating a network of detector systems; the coverage problems that may be inherent in the network owing to the large spaces involved (especially in terminals) and the concerns associated with the number and placement of the detectors; issues associated with the resolution of false alarms; and the time delay between a detection event and the initiation of a response, which may extend to hours or longer, especially for the identification of slow-acting biological threat agents.

A non-detection-based strategy could be implemented immediately with existing technologies and would not require the years of research, development, and testing that would be needed to qualify detection technologies for deployment in the air transportation environment. Although this approach would not provide protection against all threats and there would be increased costs—for example, for improved filtration systems and increased security—implementation could be stepwise, and costs would likely be much lower than for detection-based strategies.[13] Costs might also be offset to some extent by the ancillary economic benefits of cleaner air; in fact, it is conceivable that airports and/or airlines that advertise the provision of "clean air" might enjoy a competitive advantage.

In an attack involving a fast-acting agent, the occurrence of the attack per se would not be in doubt, and a strategy using videocamera surveillance coupled with pattern-recognition software could allow for a more rapid response than could a technological detection-based strategy. To identify the specific agent used in an attack, specialized equipment could be brought to the attack site as part of the initial response. In other words, a technological sensor-based strategy has no apparent advantage over a visual observation-based strategy for an attack involving a fast-acting agent; in fact, a surveillance camera will "detect" a much broader range of toxic substance releases. Its specificity is defined in terms of acute toxicity rather than in terms of a predetermined list of anticipated chemical agents.

In the case of an attack involving a slow-acting agent, the non-detection-based strategy would begin to mitigate the impact of the attack immediately by continuously removing biological aerosol particles from the air, as illustrated in Figure 3-4. This approach would bypass the response time delay of a detection-based approach associated with a biological assay, alarm resolution, and response decision making.

Neither strategy would prevent the exposure of individuals in the immediate vicinity of the agent release site;[14] however, in the non-detection-based strategy, there may be no recognition that an attack has occurred until days later when victims begin to exhibit symptoms. By then, exposed individuals would be geographically dispersed, and it would take considerable time to connect the cases forensically to an initial exposure point.[15] With no early indication that an attack had occurred, there would be no means of locating and isolating the release point so as to prevent further exposures as passenger traffic through the site continued.

In the scenario involving slow-acting agent, the detection-based strategy offers significant benefits: even if the detection of an attack and the identification of the agent used took an hour or more, action could still be taken to notify and pretreat exposed individuals while they were still in the vicinity, prevent new exposures from occurring, remediate the site, and initiate a forensic investigation. Thus, in terms of mitigating the impact of an attack with a slow-acting agent, the early detection and identification of agent and continuous air-treatment approaches could be complementary.

SUMMARY

Each of the defensive strategies discussed in this chapter—the detection-based strategy and the non-detection-based strategy—has strengths and weaknesses in protecting U.S. air transportation spaces from terrorist attack with chemical/biological agents. The non-detection-based strategy has several undeniable advantages—it is cheaper, has a faster initial response, is more robust with respect to a wide variety of potential threat agents, and can be implemented now. Thus, combined with improved video surveillance, it represents a reasonable baseline defensive strategy for protecting U.S. transportation spaces against chemical/biological attacks.

In the scenario in which an attack is perpetrated with a slow-acting biological agent, the detection-based strategy has some added benefits, particularly if the agent detection and identification time can be reduced to less than 1 hour. For this reason, developments in detector-system technology bear watching, and, if systems become reliable and cheap enough, consideration should be given to deploying them along with the baseline air-treatment systems to counter this threat. Owing to the smaller, more controlled air volumes involved, it is likely that both detection and air-treat-

[13]Evaluating costs (and benefits) and making the comparisons among alternative approaches must be an integral part of the process of selecting specific means and strategies, but such comparisons are beyond the scope of this report.

[14]In cases in which significant air currents are present, the agent may spread throughout a large portion of the facility in a short time, even without the involvement of the HVAC system, and a large number of people may become exposed.

[15]By retaining passenger manifests and using appropriate computer algorithms, airlines may be able to work with public health professionals to track geographically dispersed outbreaks of symptoms back to a common origin. This capability would enable the direct notification of passengers who might have been exposed, which would be more effective (and cause less public alarm) than general news media announcements.

ment systems will be technically feasible for the protection of aircraft before they become feasible for the protection of airport terminals.

The costs and benefits of both strategies could be evaluated more easily if models could be developed to simulate the spread of chemical/biological agents released under various scenarios in various transportation spaces, as well as their removal or neutralization via continuous treatment technologies. The committee's recommendations for the roles and responsibilities of government agencies in developing these models and its recommendations for exploring these defensive strategies are discussed in the next chapter.

4

Implementation of Defensive Strategies: The Role of the Transportation Security Administration

This chapter briefly outlines some of the current institutional and programmatic responses of government agencies, universities, and private industry to the threat posed by terrorist attacks using chemical/biological agents. It also presents the committee's findings and recommendations regarding the role that the Transportation Security Administration (TSA) should play in defending the U.S. air transportation system against such attacks.

CURRENT GOVERNMENT RESPONSE TO THE CHEMICAL/BIOLOGICAL THREAT

Many federal agencies are actively involved in both funding and conducting research to develop defensive strategies and technologies for dealing with chemical/biological threats. These agencies include the Department of Defense (DOD), the Department of Energy's (DOE's) national laboratories, the Department of Homeland Security (DHS), the National Science Foundation (NSF), the Centers for Disease Control and Prevention, and many others. Interagency groups such as the Technical Support Working Group (TSWG) have also been formed to solicit ideas for solving homeland security problems and to provide grants for further research.

Relevant Agency Programs and Resources

The committee reviewed several federal chemical/biological research programs that appeared to have application to the U.S. air transportation environment. Two programs that are perhaps most relevant in this context are the Program for Response Options and Technology Enhancements for Chemical/Biological Terrorism (PROTECT) and Protective and Response Options for Airport Counter-Terrorism (PROACT). These programs, which originated in the late 1990s under DOE's Chemical and Biological National Security Program, focus on the protection of transportation facilities against chemical/biological attacks. Partnerships to protect subway systems—and later, airports—began under PROTECT, and these programs later diverged, with subway work continuing under PROTECT and airport work shifting to PROACT. PROACT is now funded by DHS.

Under PROTECT, the subway system in Washington, D.C., has been a focus for tests involving the use of sensor technology to detect chemical agents; about half of the city's underground stations have been outfitted with chemical sensors.[1] PROACT has focused on a collaboration with the San Francisco International Airport (SFIA) to determine how threat agent simulants[2] released into the air in various airport spaces would spread and to assess what air-handling and evacuation response strategies would be most effective in limiting exposures of airport patrons.[3,4] As part of this effort, a war-game-type exercise was held in November 2003, that brought together key airport authorities and local decision makers to explore how response decisions would be made during a real attack.[5] The exercise showed the difficulty of developing an effective and timely response to a threat that cuts across so many diverse jurisdictions and areas of responsibility (airport operations, security, fire con-

[1]"Spain Blast Prompts Demands for Funds," *Washington Post*, March 22, 2004, p. B5.

[2]Theatrical smoke was used to simulate threat aerosols, and the gas SF_6 was used to simulate chemical agents.

[3]*Tracer Release Experiments at San Francisco International Airport to Improve Preparedness Against Chemical and Biological Terrorism*, Sandia Report SAND2001-8380, Albuquerque, N.Mex.: Sandia National Laboratories, June 2001.

[4]*Assessments of San Francisco International Airport to Improve Preparedness Against Chemical and Biological Terrorism*, Sandia Report SAND2003-8554, Albuquerque, N.Mex.: Sandia National Laboratories, September 2003.

[5]*Summary of the 2003 San Francisco International Airport Bio-Defense Preparedness Exercise*, Sandia Report SAND2004-2225, Albuquerque, N.Mex.: Sandia National Laboratories, May 2003.

trol and prevention, public health and safety, environment, and so on) and illustrated the importance of having response plans in place ahead of time with clearly defined roles for the relevant actors. The PROACT program has published a guidance document that draws together the lessons learned from the collaboration with SFIA to help other airports develop response plans to counter future chemical/biological attacks.[6]

Guidance is also available from a number of government sources on steps that building owners or managers can take to help protect occupants from airborne chemical, biological, or radiological attacks,[7] and on how they can choose the most appropriate air filtration and/or cleaning systems.[8] The Defense Advanced Research Projects Agency (DARPA) has had an Immune Building Program under way for several years to develop effective strategies for protecting military buildings from chemical/biological attacks. The DARPA program had the goal of developing an integrated set of models and analysis tools to help users understand the vulnerabilities of their buildings and to predict the performance of various defensive architectures. However, DARPA has found that theoretical models are not sufficient; rather, empirical testing in full-scale building areas is essential for addressing these issues with confidence.[9] The committee notes that the options and procedures available for the protection of the occupants of military buildings may be rather different from those available for protecting civilian spaces such as airport terminals.

Ongoing Research and Development Programs

The committee received briefings that provided an overview of the very large number of research efforts to develop detection technologies (Figure 4-1) and of the range of specific technology approaches (Figure 4-2) being investigated. The Department of Defense (DOD) has provided much of the funding for current systems, and DOD has fielded a number of detector prototypes as indicated in Figure 4-1. Near-term research is also being funded by the Department of Energy (DOE), Department of Homeland Security (DHS), Defense Threat Reduction Agency, and TSWG, whereas longer-term projects are being funded by DARPA, the Soldier Biological and Chemical Command (SBCCOM), Naval Research Laboratory, Army Research Laboratory, and National Science Foundation (NSF).

In a previous report,[10] this committee evaluated one of the technologies cited in Figure 4-2—mass spectrometry—for its potential to improve on current capabilities to detect trace quantities of explosives, chemical agents, and biological agents that might adhere to potential terrorists or their luggage. Another National Research Council (NRC) committee evaluated a wide range of technologies for their potential to rapidly detect and/or identify biological agents.[11] That committee found that within the next 10 years, a number of promising detection systems should become available that can substantially improve the defenses of high-value buildings and extended military bases against chemical/biological attacks. Nevertheless, on the basis of its earlier work on mass spectrometry, the wide range of presentations made to the committee by various technology analysts, and the expertise of its current members, it is this committee's judgment that, although there is great potential for several of these technologies in the future, there is currently no detection system that can operate for long periods of time and reliably detect a wide range of agents in an airport context with few false alarms.

THE ROLE OF THE TRANSPORTATION SECURITY ADMINISTRATION

Despite widespread recognition that the U.S. air transportation system remains an attractive target for terrorists to attack with chemical/biological agents and despite the large federal investment in detection technologies, no federal agency has been assigned clear responsibility for the defense of U.S. air transportation spaces against such an attack. Although some preliminary studies have considered various threat scenarios and contingency plans, at this writing these studies have involved a limited number of spaces[12] within a

---

[6]*Guidance to Improve Airport Preparedness Against Chemical and Biological Terrorism,* Version 2.1, Sandia Report SAND2005-0145, Albuquerque, N.Mex.: Sandia National Laboratories, February 2005.

[7]See, for example, *Guidance for Protecting Building Environments from Airborne Chemical, Biological, or Radiological Attacks*, Department of Health and Human Services (NIOSH) Pub. No. 2002-139, May 2002, and references therein. Available online at http://www.cdc.gov/niosh/bldvent/2002-139B.html. Accessed October 12, 2005.

[8]*Guidance for Filtration and Air Cleaning Systems to Protect Building Environments from Airborne Chemical, Biological, or Radiological Attacks,* Department of Health and Human Services (NIOSH) Pub. No. 2003-136, April 2003. Available online at http://www.cdc.gov/niosh/docs/2003-136/2003-136b.html. Accessed October 12, 2005.

[9]A variety of documents describing the DARPA Immune Building Program can be found at http://www.DARPA.mil, and http://www.natick.army.mil/soldier/JOCOTAS/ColPro_Papers/Alving.pdf. Accessed October 12, 2005.

[10]National Research Council, *Opportunities to Improve Airport Passenger Screening with Mass Spectrometry,* Washington, D.C.: The National Academies Press, 2004.

[11]National Research Council, *Sensor Systems for Biological Agent Attacks: Protecting Buildings and Military Bases*, Washington, D.C.: The National Academies Press, 2005. This committee has not attempted to improve on this discussion by trying to predict when (or if) the specific technologies mentioned in Figure 4-2 in this chapter might become commercially available.

[12]For example, attacks within an aircraft itself have not been considered under PROACT.

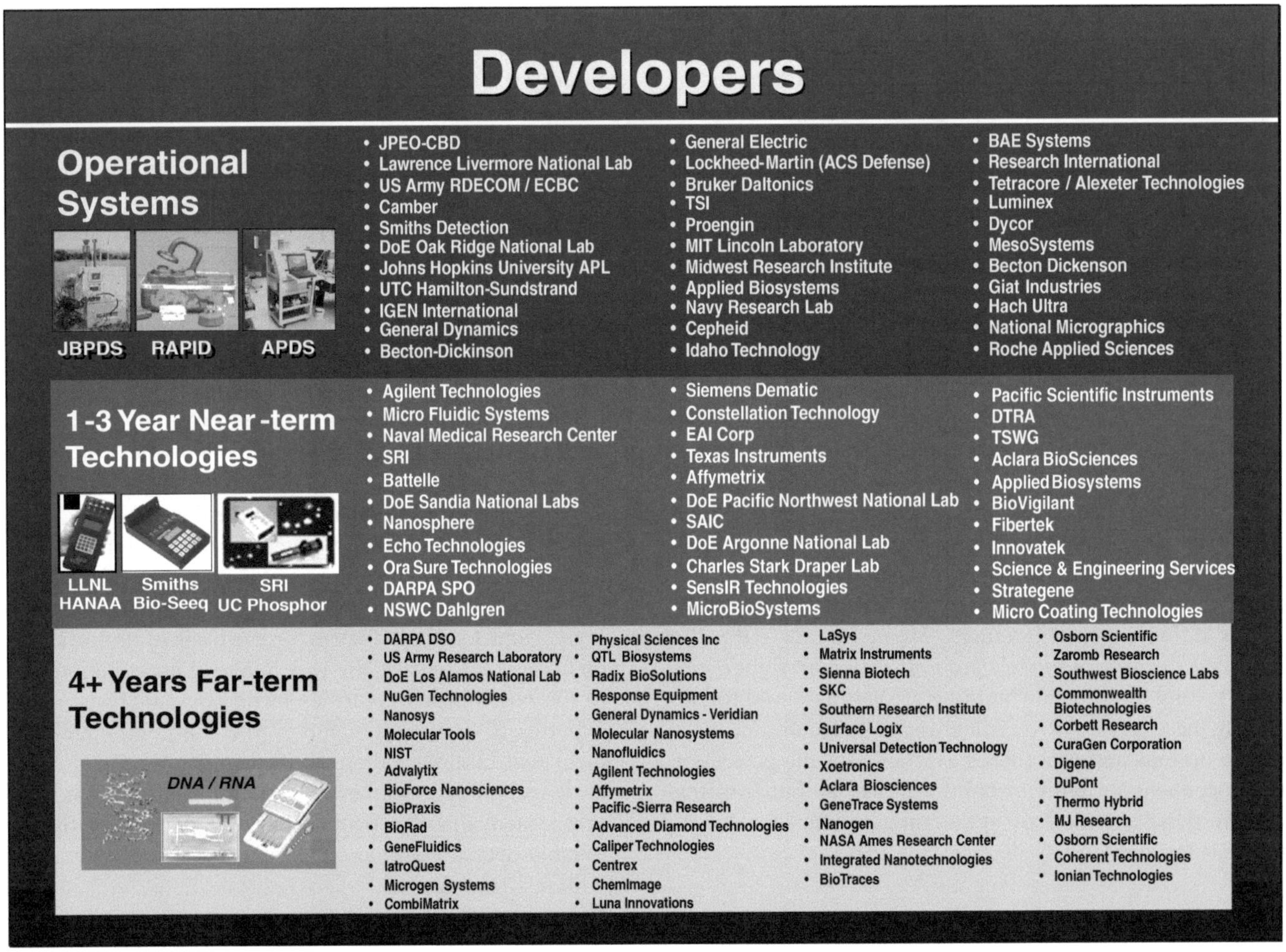

FIGURE 4-1 Partial list of chemical/biological detection system developers. NOTE: JBPDS, Joint Biological Point Detection System; RAPID, Ruggedized Advanced Pathogen Identification Device; APDS, Autonomous Pathogen Detection System; LLNL, Lawrence Livermore National Laboratory; HANAA, Handheld Advanced Nucleic Acid Analyzer; SRI, SRI International; UC, Upconverting. SOURCE: Briefing presented to the committee by Thomas Austin, Boeing Phantom Works, Woods Hole, Massachusetts, October 14, 2003.

single airport (SFIA). Clearly, much remains to be done to expand this effort and to encourage airports across the country to assess the threat and develop defensive architectures that make sense for their own particular facilities.

Finding 1: The U.S. air transportation system is an attractive target for attacks with chemical or biological weapons, yet no federal agency has been assigned clear responsibility for developing a strategy for defense against such attacks.

Based on its recent experience in facilitating the deployment of explosives-detection equipment at airports around the country, DHS's Transportation Security Administration (TSA) has established relationships with local airport authorities and is the agency most knowledgeable about U.S. air transportation spaces. It is therefore well positioned to contribute to helping airports develop defenses against chemical/biological threats.[13]

Recommendation 1: The Transportation Security Administration, with its responsibility for the federal oversight of security operations at U.S. airports, should integrate strategies for defense against chemical/biological attacks into its broader security plan for protecting the U.S. air transportation system. The line of authority and accountability for implementing these strategies should be clearly defined.

[13]The federal security directors at all major airports (these individuals are TSA employees) have operational control for security and are charged with organizing and implementing crisis management response plans.

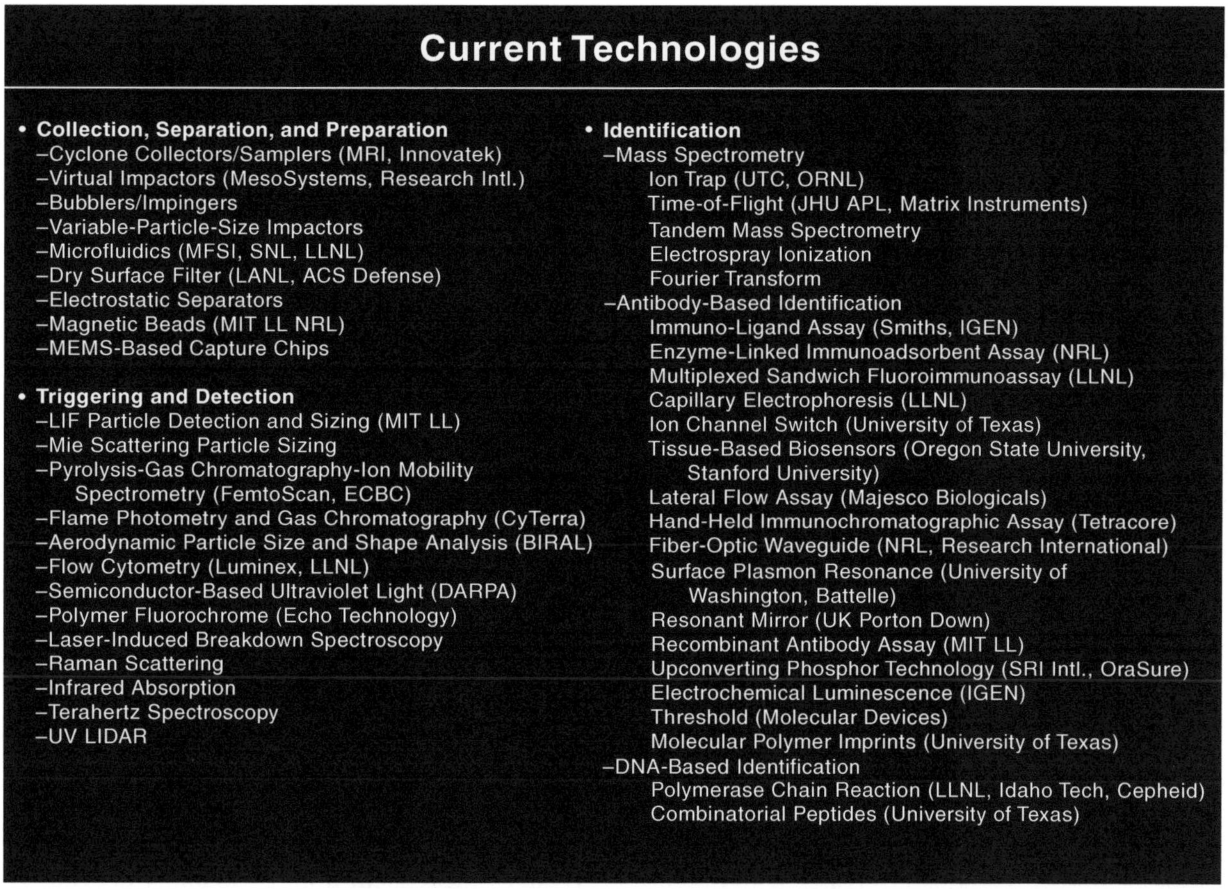

FIGURE 4-2 Partial list of technologies being investigated for various stages of chemical/biological detection systems. NOTE: MEMS, microelectromechanical systems; LIF, laser-induced fluorescence; UV LIDAR, ultraviolet light detection and ranging. SOURCE: Briefing presented to the committee by Thomas Austin, Boeing Phantom Works, Woods Hole, Massachusetts, October 14, 2003.

The committee does not suggest that TSA should be given a lead role in the development of chemical/biological-detection technologies, nor should it attempt to duplicate other agencies' programs. However, TSA can be assigned a coordinating and oversight role in the development and implementation of defensive strategies for transportation spaces.

Finding 2: No specific strategies, approaches, or procedures have been developed to defend the U.S. air transportation system against chemical/biological attacks.

The Department of Homeland Security has funded preliminary studies to elaborate specific chemical/biological threat vectors and to increase understanding of airflows in several terminals and boarding areas of San Francisco International Airport and Albuquerque Airport. It has also conducted an exercise in which the many airport decision makers (e.g., in areas of operations, security, fire control and prevention, public health and safety, and environmental issues) come together to try to formulate a coordinated response to a simulated chemical/biological attack. Such studies and exercises are valuable and should result in useful guidance that can help airports throughout the country begin to think about their own response plans. However, the work thus far is preliminary and of limited scope, and TSA itself appears to have had little involvement.

Recommendation 2: The Transportation Security Administration, in collaboration with other appropriate entities within the Department of Homeland Security,[14] should create a high-level task force to perform the following functions:

- **Create a validated threat assessment document for air transportation spaces and keep it updated;**

[14]Currently, the DHS entity with the most knowledge and experience in this area is the Science and Technology Directorate.

- **Take advantage of ongoing research aimed at the de velopment of models of the airflow within aircraft, terminals, and so forth, based on empirical studies of specific facilities, and explore the dispersal of chemical/biological simulants under various release scenarios;**
- **Create guidance to help air transportation facilities develop a threat defense strategy; and**
- **Determine unique air transportation requirements for dealing with chemical/biological threats and coordinate closely with other agencies that are active in the chemical/biological threats area to ensure that these requirements are given visibility in their programs.**

The threat assessment document should include the best intelligence on the most likely sources and sites of terrorist attacks against the system and should be updated continuously. The TSA should also build on modeling work conducted under DARPA's Immune Building Program and earlier DHS work with two airports to facilitate the development of defensive strategies and to help evaluate their efficacy. Models must include explicit consideration of the behavior of people as decision makers and as members of crowds, although research is lacking in both areas in the context of terrorism.

The TSA should build on work already being done within DHS to help airports develop an effective concept of operations for a threat defense strategy, including contingency plans for the following: scenarios involving the release of various threat agents, plans for limiting the spread of agents once released, plans for the evacuation of personnel to safe areas, plans for the isolation of contaminated areas, strategies for the early notification and treatment of potentially exposed individuals, and timely remediation of affected areas. The guidance should stress the importance of having well-defined roles and responsibilities for the many local, state, and federal authorities and airport decision makers in responding to a future attack.

The TSA should ensure that the requirements of detection systems in the transportation environment (for example, probability of detection, probability of false alarms, ruggedness, system footprint, operator interface) are considered in the relevant programs of other agencies. While TSA does participate in interagency groups that discuss homeland security issues (e.g., the Technical Support Working Group), the specific requirements of transportation systems have not been given a high priority according to briefings to the committee by TSA personnel who have attended these meetings.

Implementation of Defensive Strategies

As discussed in Chapter 3, a detection-based defensive strategy could complement the non-detection-based strategy in some scenarios, particularly those involving the release of slow-acting biological agents. However, it is likely to be some years before technological detection systems become available that are sufficiently affordable, effective, and robust for deployment in air transportation spaces.

Finding 3: Many alternative chemical/biological detection technologies are being investigated in university, industry, and government laboratories, and various military prototype systems have been developed; however, it is very difficult to independently evaluate all of the performance claims for these technologies.

A staggering number of papers is published each year in the literature on various candidate chemical/biological-detection systems. Researchers and manufacturers make diverse claims of detection limits, sensitivity, false-alarm rates, and robustness for these systems. The committee believes that in many cases, researchers emphasize the strengths of their particular detection systems while minimizing or ignoring their flaws. This practice makes it virtually impossible to evaluate the likely performance of a detection system in real-world transportation environments.

Recommendation 3: The Transportation Security Administration should keep abreast of ongoing research on chemical/biological detector technologies without starting an in-house research and development activity. Rather, it should seek to leverage the research programs of other agencies, and it should consider supporting a vendor-independent testing capability in order to verify performance claims made for chemical/biological detection systems.

The TSA has been concerned with the deployment of technologies for the detection of small arms and explosives; it has neither the resources nor the expertise to conduct its own research programs in the chemical/biological area. However, TSA's technology-monitoring effort might involve maintaining a close liaison with the efforts of other agencies, as well as funding a third party to survey the spectrum of detection technologies being developed in the private sector in order to identify those that might be most appropriate for the transportation environment.

Given the very large number of candidate detection technologies and the many (often overly optimistic) performance claims for them, TSA should also consider supporting an independent body to develop test criteria and conduct standard tests to evaluate the performance of chemical/biological detection systems and to verify the claims of prospective manufacturers. Such an independent testing body would benefit the ongoing research efforts of many government agencies.

Finding 4: Although the rapid detection of a chemical/biological attack and identification of the agent used are worthwhile objectives, a defensive strategy that depends exclusively on a detection-system alarm before action is

taken (i.e., employment of a "detect and react" strategy) has several serious limitations.

As discussed in Chapters 2 and 3, chemical/biological agent detectors can play a valuable role in defensive architectures for air transportation spaces, especially for the scenario of an attack with a delayed- or slow-acting agent. Videocamera surveillance of air transportation spaces, which can be considered a kind of functional detection technology for attacks with fast-acting agents, is available today. Technological detection systems with acceptable cost and performance are not likely to be available for some years. In the meantime, much can be done to improve the defenses of transportation spaces by blending elements of the detection-based and non-detection-based strategies that are available today.

Recommendation 4: Given the limitations of sensor- and assay-based chemical/biological agent detection and identification technologies, the Transportation Security Administration should pursue a baseline defensive strategy against chemical/biological attacks that does not depend solely on the technological detection of threat agents to initiate action. Such a strategy would be based on elements such as the following:

- **Protective and preventative steps and enhanced security;**
- **Improved visual surveillance of air transportation spaces;**
- **The establishment of a separate air supply for spaces that have a critical function (e.g., cockpits, flight-control towers, emergency-response centers); and**
- **Continuous air treatment to neutralize and/or remove agents or contaminants.**

It is the judgment of this committee that the very large number of candidate sensor-based and assay-based detection systems have received a great deal of attention and research money but that none currently has the effectiveness, technical maturity, reliability, sensitivity, and selectivity to many different agents and the low-cost characteristics needed for deployment in the air transportation environment. In contrast, there are a variety of technologies that do not involve the detection of an agent that can prevent or mitigate the consequences of a chemical/biological attack, are available today, and would be arguably less costly to deploy. These non-technological-detector-based defensive measures have not received the attention and analysis that the committee believes they deserve.

Generally, the committee believes that technologies associated with non-detection-based strategies (e.g., air cleaning, better security, better control of airflows) are nearer term, while technologies associated with detection-based strategies (with the exception of videocamera surveillance) are longer term or more speculative. Guided by the threat defense strategy described above, TSA should work with individual airports to explore security enhancements such as limiting access to identified areas of vulnerability—for example, the inlets of the terminal heating, ventilation, and air conditioning (HVAC) systems or the ventilation system for aircraft on the ground. Using experimental testing of the dispersion of released agent simulants, TSA should also work with the facilities to explore methods for limiting the spread of chemical/biological agents once they are released, such as automatic shut down of HVAC systems balancing of adjacent air-handling regions, and so on.

To combat the threat of an attack with fast-acting agent, TSA should explore the feasibility of the widespread deployment of surveillance cameras throughout transportation spaces that would enable a monitor to quickly determine that such an attack had occurred. Such cameras could also provide a dual-use value in improving the overall security environment. The TSA should fund the creation of computer models of crowd behavior during such an attack that would enable pattern-recognition software to monitor the surveillance cameras so as to provide backup for human monitors. This software should not be seen as a stand-alone system but as part of a hybrid human/software solution that recognizes the complementary capabilities of human and machine. In addition, many critical nodes in the air transportation system (control rooms, emergency-response centers, and so on) are supplied with air that is recirculated from publicly accessible areas; this makes them vulnerable to being disabled by the release of chemical/biological agents in these public areas. Thus, it may be prudent to ensure that these critical nodes have an independent air supply and are kept at a positive pressure with respect to surrounding areas.

Finally, to mitigate the impacts of a release involving either fast- or slow-acting agents, TSA should explore the feasibility of a program to use the HVAC system in a terminal or the Environmental Control System in an aircraft to continuously treat the air in transportation spaces in order to remove harmful chemicals and biological particles. This approach could involve improved air filtration and cleaning, ultraviolet irradiation of filters to kill biological organisms, plasma cleaning of air, or other technologies that are widely used to clean the air in hospitals, biology research laboratories, and industrial clean rooms. A feasibility study would include the costs (both first cost and maintenance/replacement cost), number, and optimum placement of air-cleaning units required, their effectiveness in removing threat agents from the air under various release scenarios, the number of likely exposures prevented, and so on. Such a "clean air" approach would also likely be appealing to the traveling public that is concerned about the transmission of common diseases such as colds, flu, and even severe acute respiratory syndrome (SARS), in densely populated, enclosed transportation spaces.

In the event that chemical/biological detection systems become available with appropriate cost and performance attributes and demonstrated benefits for defending against the attack scenarios of interest, TSA should consider deploying them to augment the effectiveness of the baseline non-detection-based strategy.

CONCLUSION

It appears that, given the need to maintain convenient public access to an efficient transportation system, a terrorist attack on the system with chemical/biological agents would be difficult to prevent and would likely result in a significant number of casualties. Because there are a very large number of possible chemical and biological agents that might be used in a future terrorist attack, and because the specific type of agent to be used will not, in general, be known in advance, the development and deployment of chemical sensors and bioassays for arbitrarily selected specific agents offer little real protection. By contrast, the deployment of video monitors and/or biology-based "functional" detectors (analogous to the canary in the mine) that indicate the effects of any fast-acting toxic chemical agents would be beneficial in some attack scenarios, and these systems could be deployed in a complementary way with non-detection-based defensive strategies. Thus, the overall impact of such an attack may depend less on the development of technologies for the detection of threat agents than on prudent protective measures that can be implemented *before the attack ever takes place.* The TSA should explore the feasibility of these options and should help local authorities and facilities develop contingency plans for responding to chemical/biological attacks on the U.S. air transportation system.

Appendix

Biographies of Committee Members

James F. O'Bryon, *Chair*, served as deputy assistant secretary of defense until his retirement in 2001. During his 15 years at the Pentagon, he served under seven secretaries of defense as director, Live Fire Testing, and deputy director, Operational Test and Evaluation. Mr. O'Bryon also worked in various positions within the Office of the Director, Defense Research and Engineering in the Office of the Undersecretary of Defense for Acquisition and Technology, overseeing and directing test and evaluation activities for the Secretary of Defense. These activities included the examination of the test plan adequacy, test execution, and vulnerability, lethality, and survivability of the nation's major defense systems, and the application of tactics and doctrine to these issues. He has testified before various committees of the U.S. Congress on defense and homeland security issues as well as drafting the Secretary of Defense's reports on system survivability, vulnerability, and lethality. He has served on more than a dozen committees addressing such issues as directed energy, ozone-depleting compounds, and modeling and simulation. His degrees are from the King's College, George Washington University, and the Massachusetts Institute of Technology. Mr. O'Bryon has also served for nearly 20 years as a mathematician, ballistician, and weapons systems analyst at the Ballistic Research Laboratories and the Army's Materiel Systems Analysis Activity. He currently works as an independent defense consultant for several government entities, not-for-profit organizations, and defense industries and serves as president of The O'Bryon Group.

Sandra L. Hyland, *Vice Chair*, is Etching System group manager, Tokyo Electron (TEL) Technology Center, America, responsible for TEL's etch process development at SUNY Albany's Nanotechnology Center. She supports oxide and low-k film etch for integrated development projects for TEL and IBM, as well as for other members of the Nanotechnology Center. Dr. Hyland was formerly East Coast manager for TEL Etch Systems, analyzing technology trends and customer data to determine hardware and process needs for manufacturing current and next-generation computer chips, including both capability and cost-reduction considerations. She had previously been an integration engineer for IBM's radiation-hardened computer chip manufacturing facility and had managed a processing facility for the Jet Propulsion Laboratory to assess various materials for their potential as solar-cell substrates. Dr. Hyland was also a staff officer for the National Research Council's (NRC's) National Materials Advisory Board, where she managed committees on aviation security and the design of U.S. paper money. She has a Ph.D. in materials science from Cornell University and an M.S. and a B.S. in electrical engineering from Rutgers, the State University of New Jersey, and Rensselaer Polytechnic Institute, respectively.

Cheryl A. Bitner is program director for Electronic Warfare Trainers, Maintenance Trainers, Gunnery System Trainers, and On-Board (Embedded) Trainers at AAI Corporation. She has more than 21 years of industry experience in providing training and simulation products for government as well as commercial customers, and has a strong background in cost- and schedule-control techniques. Her responsibilities include ensuring positive program performance, strategic planning, and personnel management and development. Ms. Bitner is a certified project management professional and is a member of the National Training and Simulation Association. She has published a cost-and-benefit analysis of piloting and navigational team trainers and contributes to the *AAI Training Systems Newsletter*. Ms. Bitner completed the advanced program management course at the Defense Systems Management College in 1989 and holds an M.S. in engineering science and a B.S. in computer science from Loyola College.

Donald E. Brown is chair of the Department of Systems Engineering of the University of Virginia. His research focuses on data fusion and simulation optimization, with applications to intelligence, security, logistics, and transportation. He has developed decision-support systems for several U.S. intelligence agencies and was previously an intelligence operations officer for the U.S. Army. Dr. Brown is coeditor of *Operations Research and Artificial Intelligence: The Integration of Problem Solving Strategies* (Kluwer Academic Publishers, 1990) and *Intelligent Scheduling Systems* (Kluwer, 1995) and is an associate editor for the journal *International Abstracts in Operations Research.* He has been president, vice president, and secretary of the Systems, Man, and Cybernetics Society of the Institute of Electrical and Electronics Engineers. He is past chair of the Technical Section on Artificial Intelligence of the Institute for Operations Research and Management Science and was awarded that society's outstanding service award.

John B. Daly recently retired from the U.S. Department of Transportation (DOT). He worked in the Office of Intelligence and Security (OIS) and was part of the immediate staff of the secretary of transportation, from the inception of the OIS in 1990 in the aftermath of the terrorist attack on Pan Am 103, and he served as the associate director for security policy from 1994 until his retirement. From the beginning of Mr. Daly's work in OIS, security research and development has been a major focus of his work, particularly that involving explosives and weapons detection. He is the founding chair of the Gordon Research Conference on Illicit Substance Detection, which meets annually to review and stimulate research at the frontiers of science and national policy on the detection of explosives, narcotics, and chemical/biological agents. He is the founding chair of the Transportation Security Experts Group in the Asia-Pacific Economic Cooperation's Transportation Working Group (TPT-WG); this group was established in 2000 at the 18th meeting of the TPT-WG in Miyazaki, Japan, to address security in all modes of transportation—land, sea, and air. The press of events, however, has focused its work thus far primarily on aviation security. From 1975 to 1990, he worked for the U.S. Coast Guard in strategic planning for the enforcement of laws and treaties, dealing primarily with the interdiction of drugs and illegal aliens, rising to be chief of the Plans and Policies Branch in the Office of the Chief of Staff. Mr. Daly received a B.S. from Georgetown University's School of Foreign Service, a master's degree from the University of Southern California's School of Public Administration, and a graduate diploma in naval warfare from the U.S. Naval War College.

Colin G. Drury is professor of industrial engineering at the State University of New York at Buffalo and executive director of the Center for Industrial Effectiveness, where he has worked extensively in the integration of ergonomics/human factors into company operations. His efforts have resulted in increased competitiveness and job growth for regional industry and in his receipt of two National Association of Management and Technical Assistance Centers' Project of the Year awards. Since 1990, Dr. Drury has headed a team applying human factors to the inspection and maintenance of civil aircraft, with the goal being error reduction. He performed a study for the Air Transport Association evaluating the FAA's modular bomb set and the use of this bomb set in training and testing security screeners. Dr. Drury is a fellow of the Human Factors and Ergonomics Society, the Institute of Industrial Engineers, and the Ergonomics Society. In 1981 he was awarded the Bartlett Medal by the Ergonomics Society, and in 1992 the Paul Fitts Award by the Human Factors and Ergonomics Society. He has a Ph.D. in production engineering from Birmingham University, specializing in work design and ergonomics.

Patrick Griffin is a senior member of the technical staff at Sandia National Laboratories and was chair of the NRC Panel on Assessment of Practicality of Pulsed Fast Neutron Analysis for Aviation Security. He possesses extensive expertise in the area of radiation technology. At Sandia National Laboratories, Dr. Griffin performs research in the areas of radiation modeling and simulation, neutron effects testing, radiation dosimetry, and radiation damage to materials. He is active in the standardization community and is the current chair of the American Society of Testing and Materials (ASTM) Subcommittee E10.05 on Nuclear Radiation Metrology.

Jiri (Art) Janata is professor of chemistry at the Georgia Institute of Technology. He has broad experience and expertise in the area of chemical sensors. He was previously associate director for materials and interfaces in the Environmental Molecular Science Laboratory at the Pacific Northwest National Laboratory. His research areas include analytical chemistry, electrochemistry, chemical sensors, bioinstrumentation, biophysical chemistry, fundamentals of materials science, micromachining, and instrumental analysis. Professor Janata has organized and chaired numerous symposia and conferences in his field, including Gordon Research Conferences on electrochemistry (January 1995), nuclear waste and energy (September 1996), and Chemical Sensors and Interfacial Design (July 1998). He is on the editorial boards of three journals: *Biosensors; Sensor Technology;* and *Talanta.* He is on the advisory board of *Analytical Chemistry* and is associate editor for *Field Analytical Chemistry and Technology.* Professor Janata has received numerous awards for his research (Alexander von Humboldt Senior Scientist Prize, 1987; Outstanding Research Award, University of Utah, 1990 (declined); Heyrovsky Medal, Czechoslovak Academy of Sciences, 1990; finalist medal, "Science pour l'Art 1992," Moet Hennessy and Louis Vuitton, 1992; and outstanding achievement award, Electrochemical Society, October 1994). He has been a visiting professor at many outstanding universities around the world (Wolfson College, Oxford

University, 1986/1987; Ecole Polytechnique Federale de Lausanne, 1990; and Tokyo Institute of Technology, 1995).

Harry E. Martz, Jr., is area leader for the nondestructive evaluation research and development thrust for the Lawrence Livermore National Laboratory. He has experience in explosives-detection systems and served as a member of the NRC Committee on Commercial Aviation Security. Dr. Martz has extensive background in the use of computed tomography and x-ray radiography (technologies commonly used in explosives detection) to perform nondestructive evaluation. His current projects include the use of nonintrusive x- and gamma-ray computed tomography techniques as three-dimensional imaging tools for understanding material properties and assaying radioactive waste forms. Dr. Martz has served on several NRC committees and panels dealing with the general topic of aviation security. In addition, he chaired the NRC Panel on Technical Regulation of Explosives Detection Systems.

Richard McGee is a retired electronics engineer with 35 years at the Ballistic/Army Research Laboratory (ARL), Aberdeen Proving Ground, Maryland, currently working part-time as a senior scientist contractor at ARL. Mr. McGee possesses strong engineering skills and experience in advanced sensor technologies. He has extensive expertise in millimeter-wave, infrared, radiometry, radar, smart munitions, and sensor-based systems engineering and integration. He also possesses solid understanding of the procedures and tasks required to transfer technology from the research laboratory to the field. Mr. McGee has conducted field experiments to characterize near-Earth propagation of millimeter waves (10 mm to 1 mm wavelength) in turbid and tactically hostile environments. He has designed, fabricated, and field-tested brassboard smart munitions sensors and has designed and fabricated instrumentation to measure millimeter radiometric and radar signatures of red and blue combat vehicles and signatures of various terrains. He has worked on projects involving microwave and millimeter-wave holography, development of multispectral fusion target recognition algorithms, and Synthetic Aperture Radar and Inverse Synthetic Aperture Radar high-resolution instrumentation (3.2 mm and 2.2 mm). Mr. McGee is highly skilled in systems integration and engineering for smart munitions, with a working knowledge of sensors, warheads, guidance and control, aerodynamics, lethality performance analysis, and high-acceleration survivability.

Richard L. Rowe is retired chief executive officer of MCMS, Inc., a $550 million electronics contract manufacturing company. His experience includes sensor technologies applied to aviation security, and his expertise includes new technologies in optics and radio frequency, electronic sensors, and switch products. He has more than 20 years of experience in the electronic sensors and switch products industry. Prior to his work in the electronics industry, Mr. Rowe was with the U.S. Army for 6 years. He has a master's degree in engineering administration from the George Washington University and a bachelor's degree in engineering and applied sciences from the U.S. Military Academy, West Point, New York. He has served on the boards of various electronics industries and was awarded the Honeywell Lund Award (a major leadership award) in 1987.

Eric R. Schwartz is director of Advanced Vehicle Systems Technology, Phantom Works at the Boeing Company. In this role he leads research and development (R&D) activities for advanced commercial and military aerospace vehicle systems and subsystems. These activities include technology development for crew systems, vehicle systems, flight management systems, software integration, and subsystems. He is also responsible for aviation security technologies such as chemical/biological threat detection/mitigation and aircraft protection. Mr. Schwartz has experience in threat analysis, bomb-blast effects, and blast testing of hardened luggage containers. He has performed Boeing and National Transportation Safety Board investigations and managed engineering analyses on terrorist bombing events on aircraft. He is a recognized expert on the structural and systems effects of threats against commercial aircraft and has presented numerous papers to the FAA, NASA, American Institute of Aeronautics and Astronautics (AIAA), U.S. Department of Defense, and international aviation authorities. Mr. Schwartz has participated on several government committees and advisory boards, including the National Research Council's Panel on Assessment of Technologies Deployed to Improve Aviation Security. He is a member of the FAA Aviation Security R&D Advisory Committee, and he served as deputy director on the AIAA Technical Committee. He has also served on the NASA Aviation Safety Executive Council, the European JAA Future Aviation Safety Team, the International Air Transport Association Aviation Security Committee, and NATO R&D Advisory Group for Aircraft Survivability.

Michael Story is retired from Thermo Electron Corporation. He was involved in the research, design, and commercialization of mass spectrometers for 37 years, and is a co-founder of the Finnigan Corporation. He was a member of previous NRC committees on commercial aviation security (1988–1993) and chaired the Panel on Test Protocol and Performance Criteria.

H. Bruce Wallace is currently a senior staff systems engineer for ORSA Corporation, where he is an internationally recognized expert on millimeter-wave (MMW) and sub-MMW technology. He retired as a civilian employee for the Department of the Army, with which he was most recently acting as deputy and director of the Weapons and Materials Research Directorate of the Army Research Laboratory. Previous to that he spent 7 years as chief of the Radio Frequency and Electronics Division, where he was responsible for the Army's basic and applied research in radio-frequency technologies. His primary area of research involved investigating the application of MMW techniques to weapons systems. This work included studies in electronic components, atmospheric and near-Earth propagation, active and passive system designs, and high-resolution polarimetric imaging. Key outcomes from his work were the development of the Sense-and-Destroy Armor MMW sensor system, the Army's High Resolution Radar Imaging facility, which provides state-of-the-art imaging of ground platforms, and the Multifunction Radio Frequency System, which has become a key electronic component in the Army's Future Combat System. He is the author of more than 60 government and open literature publications. Mr. Wallace has served on numerous Department of Defense (DOD) and NATO panels as chair or Army lead, and as lead investigator on several trade studies of DOD radar systems and capabilities. He was also a member of two NASA review panels, providing technical and managerial review of basic research programs. He is a fellow of the IEEE Geosciences and Remote Sensing Society.